T0182133

Modern Bayesian Statistics in Clinical Research

Ton J. Cleophas • Aeilko H. Zwinderman

Modern Bayesian Statistics
in Clinical Research

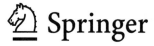 Springer

Ton J. Cleophas
Albert Schweitzer Hospital
Department Medicine Albert
Schweitzer Hospital
Sliedrecht, The Netherlands

Aeilko H. Zwinderman
Department Biostatistics and Epidemiology
Academic Medical Center Department
Biostatistics and Epidemiology
Amsterdam, Noord-Holland,
The Netherlands

Additional material to this book can be downloaded from http://extras.springer.com

ISBN 978-3-030-06507-2   ISBN 978-3-319-92747-3   (eBook)
https://doi.org/10.1007/978-3-319-92747-3

This Springer imprint is published by Springer Nature, under the registered company Springer International Publishing AG
The registered company address is: Gewerbestrasse 11, 6330 Cham, Switzerland

Preface

The current textbook has been written as a help to medical/health professionals and students for the study of modern Bayesian statistics, where posterior and prior odds have been replaced with posterior and prior likelihood distributions. Why may likelihood distributions estimate uncertainties of statistical test results better than normal distributions? Nobody knows for sure, and the use of likelihood distributions instead of normal distributions for the purpose has only just begun, but already everybody is trying and using them. SPSS statistical software version 25 (2017) has started to provide a combined module entitled Bayesian Statistics including almost all of the modern Bayesian tests (Bayesian t-tests, analysis of variance (anova), linear regression, crosstabs, etc.).

First of all, Bayesian and traditional tests are different. Bayesian tests assess whether a new treatment is better than control. Traditional tests, in contrast, test whether a new treatment is not better than control and then try and reject this null hypothesis of no difference. A number of arguments in favor of Bayesian methodologies can be given. Bayesian tests work with 95% credible intervals that are usually somewhat wider than the traditional 95% confidence intervals, and this is fine, because it may reduce the chance of statistical significances with little clinical relevance. Also, maximal likelihoods of likelihood distributions are not always identical to the mean effect of traditional tests, and this may be so, because biological likelihoods may better fit biological questions than numerical means do. In addition, Bayesian not only uses likelihood distributions but also ratios of likelihood distributions (Cauchy distributions) rather than ratios of Gaussian distributions, the latter of which are notorious for ill data fit. Fourth, Bayesian integral computations are very advanced and, therefore, give optimal precisions of complex functions and better so than traditional multiple mean calculations of nonrepresentative subsamples do. Fifth, with Bayesian testing type I and II errors need not be taken into account. Obviously, all of this sounds promising, and in the past few years, many scientists including econo-, socio-, and psychometricians are rather satisfied with the result patterns of modern Bayesian data analyses.

The authors are frequentists and know all too well that many of the above are speculative. For now we will stay modest. The advantage of Bayesian may be that a somewhat better underlying structure of your null and alternative hypotheses is given. Otherwise, it looks of course much like traditional statistics: a very small Bayes factor generally corresponds to a very small p-value. The problem for non-mathematicians is that integral calculations are needed to compute precise areas under the curve.

The current edition will begin with a brief review of the past and some explanatory chapters of modern Bayesian statistics. Then, step-by-step analyses will be given of clinical data examples according to SPSS' s recipes. Also Bayesian MCMC (Markov Chain Monte Carlo) samplings and the current search for causal relationships with Bayesian structural equation modeling will be addressed as methods where Bayesian statistics successfully helped fostering the deepest enigma of mankind, the proof of causality. We should add that each chapter can be studied as a stand-alone without the need for information from the other chapters. Both real data and hypothesized self-assessment data files are in extras.springer.com. We do hope that the current edition will be helpful to the medical and health community for which the dedication to the search for causalities is more vital than it is for most other disciplines.

Dordrecht, The Netherlands   Ton J. Cleophas
Amsterdam, The Netherlands   Aeilko H. Zwinderman

Contents

Chapter 1
General Introduction to Modern Bayesian Statistics

1.1 Background

Note: the terms chance and probability will be used as synonyms throughout this edition. With Bayesian statistics there is no traditional null (H0) and alternative hypothesis (H1) like there is with standard null hypothesis testing. Instead there is a standardized likelihood distribution to assess whether a new treatment is better or worse than control.

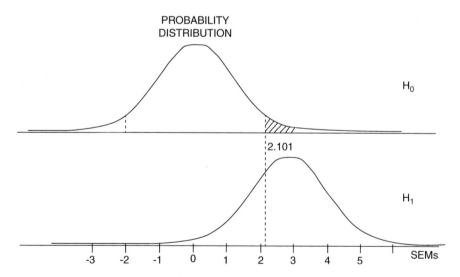

The above figure shows the graphs of traditional alternative and null hypothesis curves, H1 and H0. They are Gaussian curves with respectively mean ± standard error of the mean (SEM) and 0 ± the same standard error. If your mean > ≈2 SEMs distant from zero, like in the above graph, then we will have <5% chance to be in the

H0 area under the curve, and, therefore, we will reject H0 at p < 0.05. Bayesian and traditional tests are different. Bayesian tests assess whether a new treatment is better than control, and uses for that purpose likelihood odds or likelihood distributions of the data adjusted for prior informations if available or a noninformation factor if not. Traditional tests, in contrast, test whether a new treatment is not better than control, and then try and reject this null hypothesis of no difference. There is, however, resemblance. The Bayesian likelihood distributions often but not always support traditional H0 tests. They can be used to support powerless traditional analyses.

1.2   Introduction

Classical statistics uses the scientific method to assess whether a new treatment works or not, and it does so by trying and rejecting the null hypothesis of no effect. The classical definition of the null hypothesis is the summary of the means of many trials similar to our trial with an overall effect of zero. The scientific method is considered a gem and the "non plus ultra" for scientific research, because it is less biased than observational data, particularly if applied in prospective randomized controlled trials. However, it will only work, if you accept a number of untested assumptions, for example, that your study sample is representative for the entire population, and that we have numerous repetitions of trials and that all of them have virtually identical means and standard deviations while, in reality, we have only a single trial. Pretty strong untested assumptions include the study is representative, meaning that that if we repeat it differences will be small, and all similar studies will have the same standard deviation or error. With Bayesian statistics, there is no null hypothesis, like there is with classical statistics. Yet it can be used to estimate, whether a new treatment works or not. Estimations are done with likelihood distributions, rather than normal distributions. Why may a likelihood distribution be better than a Gaussian-like normal distribution. That is, because it runs from 0 to ∞, while the latter runs from 0 to 1 (100%). Therefore, it is mathematically better assessable, and can be added, subtracted, divided and multiplied, and even integrated and differentiated. That is exactly what we will do all the time with current Bayesian statistics. For point estimates of likelihood distributions, as routinely used in the past, odds and maximal likelihoods were used. and the same was true. They also ran from 0 to ∞ (or even −∞). Another advantage of likelihood distributions is that they are standardized. Non-standardized measures of research like means and their spread are hard to add-up, divide etc. Standardized measures such as standardized likelihood distributions of, for example, historical and current data can be divided by one another to produce a so-called Bayes factor, which is a pretty reliable estimate of evidence, that a current treatment worked better than a previous treatment did.

1.3 Traditional Bayes

Thomas Bayes from London UK, 1760, was English clergyman and mathematician / statistician who developed an interesting probability theory helpful to analyze qualitative diagnostic tests. This theory was later called Bayes' theorem:

$$\text{posterior} - \text{test odds} = \text{prior} - \text{test odds} \times \left[\,\text{sensitivity}\,/\,(1 - \text{specificity})\,\right].$$

In a population with both healthy and diseased people the accuracy of a diagnostic test is measured:

1. sensitivity is the fraction of the subjects positive tested divided by all diseased
2. specificity is the fraction of the subjects negative tested divided by all non-diseased.

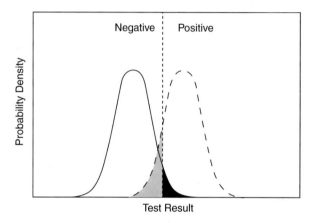

The above graph shows two Gaussian probability density curves, left are the healthy and right are the diseased subjects. Together they summarize all of the subjects included in a validation population of a qualitative test with on the x-axis individual results and on the y-axis "how often". The grey triangle are the subjects that are diseased but erroneously qualified by the test as being healthy, the black triangle are the subjects that are healthy but erroneously qualified by the test as being diseased, otherwise called the false positives. Sensitivity equals the area under the right curve right from the vertical cut-off line divided by that of the entire right curve. (1 − specificity) is the area under the left curve right from vertical cut-off divided by the entire left curve (the black triangle). The division sum of sensitivity/ (1 − specificity) is often called the likelihood ratio of sensitivity and (1 − specificity), and presents the fraction of true positive subjects from all positive subjects (also including false positive subjects). For example, with a sensitivity of 80% and a specificity of 95% of your test, you will obtain a likelihood ratio of 0.8/0.05 = 16. With equal chances of encountering disease or health you will find 16 times more often a true positive than you will find a false positive patient.

1.4   Odds and Probabilities

The odds of having a disease is not the probability, but it is closely related to it, yet somewhat hard to understand. The probability of having a disease equals in a population the number of patients with the disease divided by the entire population (a/(a + b)). It is synonymous to the chance, proportion, percentage. The odds of having a disease equals the number of patients with the disease divided by the number of patients without the disease (a/b).

disease	yes	no
	a	b

In the above population of (a + b) patients, (a/(a + b)) is the probability of having the disease, while (a/b) is the odds of having a disease. Probabilities are intuitively understood well. They run from 0 to 1.

For example, a proportion of

5/1000 is a probability of	0.005
500/1000	0.5
900/1000	0.9.

Odds of above proportions are quite different:

5/1000 gives an odds of	5/995 = 0.005025 ≈ 0.005
500/1000	500/500 = 1
900/1000	900/100 = 9.

This means that small probabilities are virtually equal to odds values. However, large probabilities are very different from their odds values. Odds run from 0 to ∞ (infinity).

Odds are pretty counterintuitive. Yet they are frequently used in statistics. This is because software programs using odds have a much better performance than those using probabilities. Fortunately, small proportions of probabilities and odds and produce virtually the same, and the interpretation of odds is generally in terms of probability. Odds plays a key role not only in logistic regressions and Cox regressions, but also in Bayes statistical analyses as post-test odds and pre-test odds

1.5   Posterior- and Prior-Test Odds

Now, this approach to identifying true positives works fine as long as we have equal chance of disease or not in your study population. However, if the prevalence of disease in your study population is only 20%, then your chance of a positive outcome is much smaller and that of a true positive patients is equally so, despite your likelihood ratio of 16. A 20 % prevalence means (with a population of 100) a prior odds of disease of $20/80 = 1/4$ instead of $50/50 = 1$. Your study outcome will change correspondingly:

$$\text{post test odds} = \text{prior test odds} \times \text{likelihood ratio}$$
$$= 1/4 \times 16$$
$$= 4.$$

This would mean that your odds of a true positive patient is only four times better rather than 16 times better. This gives a probability of $4/(1 + 4) = 0.800$ of your positive test being true positive, instead of $16/17 = 0.941$. Considering the larger odds of no disease in your study sample of 75%, it is remarkable, that its influence on the posterior odds of disease is limited: posterior probability 80% instead of 94%. Yet, you may reason, that the above Bayesian computation answers a much more important scientific question than the traditional sensitivity specificity assessment does. This is because, if your test is positive, it tells you who will really have the disease. This will often be far less than 100%. The Bayesian equation is not only applied with qualitative diagnostic tests but also and even more so with genetic research. A nice thing with genetic research is the presence of accurate prior probabilities of a disease based on Mendelian genetics precisely predicting gene carrier-ship.

In the past decade or two Bayes has come to being used with clinical research. Particularly, the question in what fraction of experiments with statistically significant results is the rejected null hypothesis really true? With drug screening the prior probability may, for example, be an expected efficacy percentage. In the next three chapters examples will subsequently be given of Bayesian analyses of diagnostic tests, of genetic research, and of drug screening. In the Chaps. 3–14 novel developments will be reviewed. Traditional Bayes works with BFs (Bayes factors), which is an invariant estimator of the ratio between the prior and posterior odds of a disease, a treatment efficacy, or any other outcome variable expressed as an odds. With modern Bayesian statistics, the invariant Bayes factor, based on a likelihood ratio of prior and the posterior likelihood odds have been replaced with a ratio of likelihood *distributions,* that have, in addition to maximal likelihoods, distributions of likelihoods.

1.6 Modern Bayes

The traditional analytic tests for null hypothesis (H0) testing compute spread in the data, otherwise called uncertainty, with the help of normal or t probability-distributions. These probability distributions are symmetric, and can be approximated from the equation

$$f(x) = \frac{1}{\sqrt{2\pi s^2}} e^{-(x-m)^2/2s^2}$$

where s = standard error and m = mean (or, with events, proportion of patients with an event).

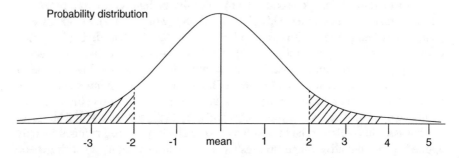

Modern Bayes does not work with normal distributions, but likelihood distributions, that are approximated differently. For continuous data they are pretty tough requiring complex integral computations. For binary data they are more easy to approximate using the binomial distribution. An example will be given. With ten trials in a test-set we have six events, proportion 6/10. According to likelihood theory, the likelihood of this outcome is not 100%. There are also likelihoods of 5, 4, 7, 9 events etc., but they are smaller than the likelihood of 6 events, because 6 is what we have actually observed, our tested data. All of the unstandardized likelihoods together add to 100%. Binomial computations are used to compute each likelihood (! indicates "faculty", for example 10! = 10 × 9 × 8.......... × 2 × 1).

$$\text{likelihood of 6 events} = \frac{10!}{6!(4!)}(0.6)^6(1-0.6)^4 = 0.26$$

$$\text{likelihood of 5 events} = \frac{10!}{6!(4!)}(0.5)^6(1-0.5)^4 = 0.21$$

$$\text{likelihood of 4 events} = \frac{10!}{6!(4!)}(0.4)^6 (1-0.4)^4 = 0.11$$

$$\text{likelihood of 3 events} = \frac{10!}{6!(4!)}(0.3)^6 (1-0.3)^4 = 0.04$$

$$\text{likelihood of 7.5 events} = \frac{10!}{6!(4!)}(0.75)^6 (1-0.75)^4 = 0.15$$

$$\text{likelihood of 8 events} = \frac{10!}{6!(4!)}(0.8)^6 (1-0.8)^4 = 0.09$$

All separate likelihoods above can be used to approach the function of the likelihood distribution from the proportion 6/10 events. A graph of this likelihood function is given underneath, with number of events theoretically possible on the x-axis, and standardized likelihoods on the y-axis. The underneath graph approximates the area under the curve of the above small sample of n = 10 events.

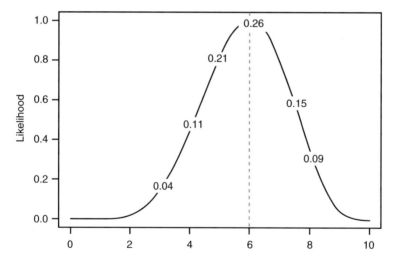

1.7   Standardized Likelihood Distributions

The graph above shows, that, although it is pretty similar to a normal distribution, it is not symmetric, and somewhat skewed to the left. If all of the separate likelihoods, as calculated above, are divided by 0.26, the largest likelihood in our example, then standardized likelihoods will be obtained, that do no longer add to $1 = 100\%$. The unit of the standardized likelihoods is the same as that of the y-axis of the above graph.

$$\text{Standardized likelihood of } 0.26 = 0.26 / 0.26 = 1.0$$

$$\text{standardized likelihood of } 0.21 = 0.21 / 0.26 = 0.82$$

$$\text{standardized likelihood of } 0.11 = 0.11 / 0.26 = 0.41$$

$$\text{standardized likelihood of } 0.04 = 0.04 / 0.26 = 0.16$$

$$\text{standardized likelihood of } 0.15 = 0.15 / 0.26 = 0.59$$

$$\text{standardized likelihood of } 0.09 = 0.09 / 0.26 = 0.35.$$

......

......

...

_____+

$$\text{The area under the curve } \left(\text{AUC}\right) \text{ of the entire}$$

$$\text{standardized likelihood distribution} \qquad \approx > 3.$$

The magnitude of this AUC is a measure of uncertainty in the data. Just like with traditional H0 testing, small samples means a pretty wide spread in the data, and, thus, much uncertainty. Also with likelihood distributions this is true. For example, the AUC of the likelihood distribution of the proportion 6/10 may be >3, while that of 60/100 reduces to close to 1. This is further explained underneath.

If instead of a sample size of 10 a sample size of 100 is taken, a likelihood distribution can be drawn and an event rate of 60 instead of 6 is observed, then similarly to the data from the above example a likelihood distribution curve can be constructed using probabilities estimated from binomial computations.

$$\text{likelihood of } 60 \text{ events} = \frac{10!}{60!(40!)}(0.6)^{60}(1-0.6)^{40} = ...$$

$$\text{likelihood of } 50 \text{ events} = \frac{10!}{60!(40!)}(0.5)^{60}(1-0.5)^{40} = ...$$

$$\text{likelihood of } 75 \text{ events} = \frac{10!}{60!(40!)}(0.75)^{60}(1-0.75)^{40} = ...$$

The standardized likelihoods are obtained as demonstrated above. For example, of

60 events it would be 1.0

50 events it would be 0.1

75 events it would be 0.0

....

....

_____+

1.1

The underneath graph gives the likelihood distribution curve.

It is much more narrow (precise) than the above curve, and this would mean, that the area under the curve of the entire likelihood distribution would be a lot smaller than it was with a sample size of only 10, namely 1.1 instead of over 3.

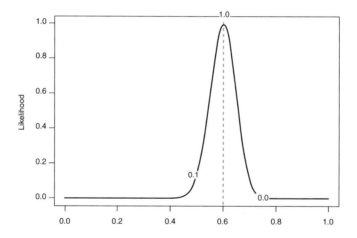

1.8 Bayes Factor

Modern Bayes works with Bayes factors. The Bayes factor is not the AUC of a likelihood distribution curve, but, rather, the ratio of the AUCs of two likelihood distributions. We should add, that the ratio of two odds values, has often been named Bayes factor with traditional Bayesian statistics, but with modern Bayesian statistics, the Bayes factors are mostly based on the ratios of two likelihood distributions. Computations of areas under the curve of nonlinear functions are required, Underneath an approximation approach is given of a nonlinear function as an example of the type of computations required. However, this is pretty imprecise, and modern software programs like SAS, SPSS, MATLAB, R, etc., routinely use integral calculations for estimating entire areas under the curve. This is pretty complicated and cannot be covered in this text, but, just to scratch the surface, some simple explanations will be given.

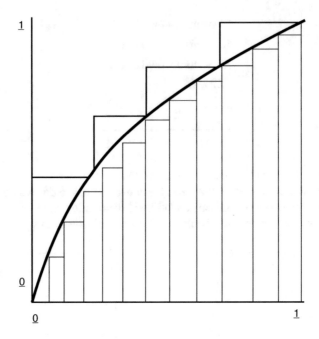

The above graph gives approximations of the nonlinear function

$$y = \sqrt{x} = x^{1/2}$$

The above approximation with 4 bars has a computed area under the curve of $\approx$ 0.73...

The above approximation with 12 bars has a computed area under the curve of $\approx$ 0.62...

The calculated integral of the function is given underneath:

$$\int_{0}^{1} x^{1/2} dx.$$

How do we proceed. All we need is the antiderivative.

The antiderivative of the function $= x^{1/2}$ equals $2/3\ x^{2/3}$.

Then, the value of the above integral can be easily computed.

It is $2/3\ (1)^{3/2} - 2/3\ (0)^{3/2} = 2/3 = 0.666666$.

It is, as expected, just in between 0.73... and 0.62....

The Bayes factor equals the ratio of the AUCs of the often nonlinear posterior and prior likelihood distribution, rather than simple functions like the above $f(x) = x^{1/2}$. Rough approximations can be obtained from graphs as will be shown in the next section, but better accuracy is obtained by integral calculations.

$$\int_{0}^{1} f(x) dx.$$

With ratios, generally, two variables, instead of one, are involved, and a trick as applied is to "integrate out" one of the two variables. This may be hard for non-mathematicians, but it is pretty straightforward. You hold one variable constant, and integrate the variable you want to get rid of. For example with the function 2/3 (x + 2y) the parameter x can be integrated out:

$$\int_{x=0}^{x=1} 2/3(x+2y)\,dx = 1/3(1+4y).$$

With probability density functions (PDFs), like likelihood distributions, you would have to take the double integral of the PDF to get a cumulative density function (CDF). Integrating out a variable from the PDF, then, gives you the AUC of the two variables, which is called the marginal density of those variables.

$$\begin{aligned}
\text{Marginal PDF}(x) &= \text{Integral } f(x,y)\,dy \\
&= \text{AUC}(y)\,\text{given } x \\
&= \text{Marginal PDF}(y) \\
&= \text{Integral}(y) \\
&= \text{Integral } f(x,y)\,dx.
\end{aligned}$$

$$\text{CDF of double integral } f(x,y)\,dxdy = \text{total AUC}.$$

Computations without the trick of integrating out may be hard. Even with it, integrals of likelihood distributions may be tough on a pocket calculator, and, fortunately, user friendly software programs have recently become available. We will use for the purpose in the current edition the Bayesian Statistics Modules in SPSS statistical software available in the advanced statistics program of version 25 (release 2017).

1.9   Uninformed Prior Likelihood Distributions, Example One

Bayesian statistics requires not only posterior distributions obtained from the measured data of your research but also prior distributions, sometimes called the Achilles heel of Bayesian analysis. Uninformative Priors, beta frequency distributions and other standardized prior likelihood distributions are an alternative to priors based on controversial prior beliefs.

It is time, that we addressed one of the flaws of traditional Bayes statistics. If you knew the prior probability, then applying Bayesian statistics would not be controversial. However, unfortunately, this is, particularly with clinical trials, rarely the case. Prior probabilities are often based on beliefs and even misbeliefs, rather than virtual certainties. So much so that they were sometimes named the bad elements of Bayesian prediction, and their parameters were named nuisance parameters. Fortunately, in the past few years clever statisticians have offered solutions. The flaw of lacking priors has been largely accounted for by adequate methodologies, including

1. the use of variance parameters from your posterior data instead,
2. the use of noninformative prior values that are equally probable in the Bayes tests used,
3. the use of prior values, that are uniform over the space relevant,
4. the use of "reference priors" (priors equal to standard beta distributions for binomial data or gamma distributions for continuous normal data),
5. the use of "conjugate priors" (priors the same as those of the posteriors as applied, however, with a standard error of 1).

We should add that, first of all, the effect of priors on the size of the Bayes factors is often pretty small (Gelman, in Encyclopedia of Environmetrics, pp 1634–7, and Berger et al. in: Likelihood methods for eliminating nuisance parameters, Stat Sci 1999; 14: 1028). Also, uninformative priors is, in fact, a contradictio in terminis. It is mostly based on something prior for example the variance, standard deviation or standard error of the posterior data. Sometimes conjugate priors are used for Bayesian computations, i.e., priors with the same likelihood distribution as those of the posteriors but with an standard error of 1. Also reference priors may be used. They are constructed from standardized beta density distributions (for binomial data) or gamma density distributions (for continuous or normal data). In many sub-sequent chapters the Bayesian versions of standard analytic models will be assessed and many types of priors will be used, and they perform pretty well. We will now give you an impression of how the Bayes factor as a ratio of two likelihood distributions, the prior and posterior, is computed, and how it can be interpreted. We will start with performing a very rough approximation method for the purpose.

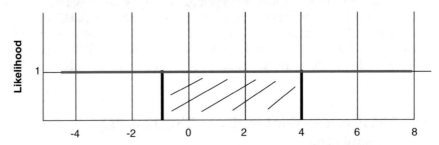

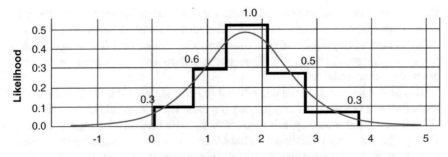

Mean: mean blood pressure reduction

The above graphs show respectively a prior and a posterior likelihood distribution of a small study of ten patients assessed for fall in mean blood pressure after treatment. The prior distribution is an example of a noninformative prior distribution of the diffuse or uniform type with function fx = 1. The graphs are redrawn and adapted from SPSS statistical software graphs. The areas under the curves (AUCs) are used to estimate the magnitude and shape likelihood distributions. Instead of exact integral calculations rough approximations are computed.

The AUC of the prior distribution is five times (from 0 to 4) those of the rectangles of $1 \times 1 = 5$.

The AUC of the posterior distribution is $0.3 \times 1 + 0.6 \times 1 + 1.0 \times 1 + 0.5 \times 1 + 0.3 \times 1 = 2.7$.

According to the Bayesian equation:

$$\text{prior likelihood distribution} \times \text{Bayes factor} = \text{posterior likelihood distribution}$$

$$5\,\text{times the rectangles} \times \text{Bayes factor} = 2.7$$

$$\text{Bayes factor} = 2.7 / 5$$

$$\approx 0.5.$$

The interpretation as compared to that of the traditional null hypothesis testing is in the underneath table copied from the Bayesian Statistics Help sheets from SPSS.

Bayes factor	Evidence category	Bayes factor	Evidence category	Bayes Factor	Evidence category
>100	Extreme evidence for H0	1–3	Anecdotal evidence for H0	1/30 to 1/10	Strong evidence for H1
30–100	Very strong evidence for H0	1	No evidence	1/100 to 1/30	Very Strong evidence for H1
10–30	Strong evidence for H0	1/3 to 1	Anecdotal evidence for H1	1/100	Extreme evidence for H1
3–10	Moderate evidence for H0	1/10 to 1/3	Moderate evidence for H1		

A Bayes factor of roughly 0.5 suggests that support for rejecting the traditional null hypothesis of no difference from zero is in the data. Also some support for the traditional H1, the alternative hypothesis (a real blood pressure reduction in the data) is observed.

1.10 Uninformed Prior Likelihood Distributions, Example Two

In a 55 patient study the number of patients responding to antihypertensive treatment are counted: the proportion of responders was 20/55. The traditional z-test assesses whether $20/55 = 0.3364$ is significantly different from 0.00. The z-value equals 5.5. It means that the proportion responders is larger than zero at p = 0.0000. The antihypertensive treatment really works. A Bayesian analysis will be performed, because of the pretty small sample of these binomial data.

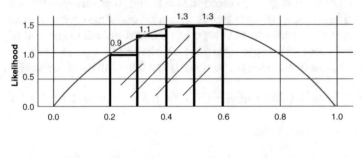

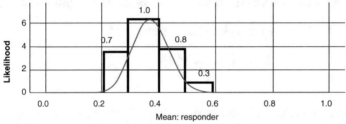

The above graphs show respectively a prior and a posterior likelihood distribution of the small study of 55 binomials. The graphs are redrawn and adapted from SPSS statistical software graphs. The areas under the curves (AUCs) are used to estimate the magnitude and shape likelihood distributions. Instead of exact integral calculations rough approximations are again used for computation.

The prior and posterior likelihood distribution curves are drawn respectively from a standard beta distribution with x = 0.5 as mean x-value, and the best fit beta distribution of the posterior data.

The areas under the curves (AUCs) are then used to estimate the magnitude and shape likelihood distributions. Instead of exact integral calculations rough approximations are computed.

Approximation of the AUC of the prior likelihood distribution
$$= 0.9 + 1.1 + 1.3 + 1.3$$
$$\approx 3$$

Approximation of the AUC of the posterior likelihood distribution
$$= 0.7 + 1 + 0.8 + 0.3$$
$$\approx 3$$

The Bayes factor $\approx 3 / 3$
$$\approx 1.$$

The interpretation as compared to that of the traditional null hypothesis testing is in the SPSS table shown in the previous section. The Bayes factor of ≈ 1 indicates that neither H0 nor H1 is supported. This result may seem disappointing considering the 0.0000 p-value of the z-test. Yet, considering the pretty small sample size of the binomial data example, it is neither entirely unrealistic.

1.11 Uninformed Prior Likelihood Distributions, Example Three

A paired samples t-test is performed of 10 patients who in a crossover study are assessed for hours of sleep after placebo or after a sleeping pill. Which of the two treatments is better. The traditional paired t-test produces a t-value of 3.184, and, thus, a p-value of 0.011. The null hypothesis of no difference is rejected. But this is a small study and we will perform a Bayesian t-test to see if we find support for the alternative hypothesis, a true difference between placebo and treatment.

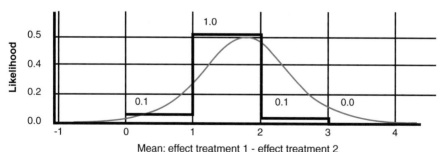

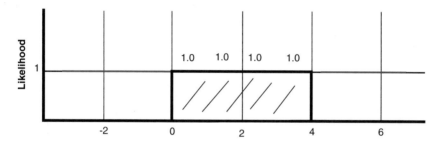

Mean: effect treatment 1 - effect treatment 2

The above graphs show respectively the prior and posterior likelihood distributions of the data from the above study in the form of a noninformative prior based on the log standard deviation of the posterior data, and a likelihood distribution of the actual data with a mean of 1.78 h and a maximal likelihood of 0.6.

Approximation of the AUC of the prior likelihood distribution

$$= 1.0 + 1.0 + 1.0 + 1.0$$

$$\approx 4$$

Approximation of the AUC of the posterior likelihood distribution

$$= 0.1 + 1.0 + 0.1 + 0.0$$

$$\approx 1.2$$

The Bayes factor $\approx 1.2 / 4$

$$\approx 0.2.$$

According to the underneath Bayes factor table, a Bayes factor of 0.2 would mean strong support for the alternative hypothesis, a true difference between placebo and sleeping pill. This result thus supports the traditional t-test result.

The examples 1–3 are more precisely assessed in the Chaps. 3–5. But this chapter is, to give you a basic understanding of prior and posterior likelihood distributions, and how they can be helpful to provide supportive evidence of a true effect in the data or not. The underneath table gives the magnitudes of the Bayes factors in support of either a traditional zero effect (above red diagonal) or an alternative effect (below red diagonal).

Reject H1

Bayes Factor	Evidence Category	Bayes Factor	Evidence Category	Bayes Factor	Evidence Category
>100	Extreme Evidence for H0	1-3	Anecdotal Evidence for H0	1/30-1/10	Strong Evidence for H1
30-100	Very Strong Evidence for H0	1	No Evidence	1/100-1/30	VeryStrong Evidence for H1
10-30	Strong Evidence for H0	1/3-1	Anecdotal Evidence for H1	1/100	Extreme Evidence for H1
3-10	Moderate Evidence for H0	1/10-1/3	Moderate Evidence for H1		

Reject H0

Section 1.7 of this chapter showed that the posterior likelihood distribution of a proportion of 6/10 (n = 10) produced an AUC of ≈ 3. The AUC of the likelihood of the same proportion with a sample size of 100 was a lot smaller, 1.1. With n = 1000 the AUC would further reduce to 1.0. With priors unchanged, obviously, a larger sample size of your study will not only produce smaller AUCs of the posterior like-lihood distributions but also smaller Bayes factors (BFs). The pattern of the above table with increasingly smaller BFs is largely due to increasing posterior data sample sizes, and will, therefore, correspondingly provide additional support in favor of the traditional alternative hypothesis.

1.12   Priors, the Achilles Heal of Modern Bayesian Statistics

In the past the non exact intuitive definition of the prior was the Achilles heal of Bayes. Fortunately, the intuitive prior and posterior odds have been replaced with more exact likelihood distributions and computations based on intervals of uncertainty. However, lacking evidence about priors still exists, and there is a whole battery of tricks to correct for it.

First, even with odds we already observed that the effect of prior on posterior is generally pretty small. With current likelihood distributions this seems to be equally true. Largely non-informative priors of different scales and shapes and even non-sense priors seem to go together with posteriors leading to adequate results, at least results comparable with those of traditional tests.

Three types of noninformative priors are being used as explained by Gelman (Prior Distribution, in: Encyclopedia of Environmetrics, Wiley Chichester 2002).

1. Noninformative priors based on uniform graphs that can be conveniently integrated out or a priori described as a simplified function of $f = 1$.
2. Conjugate priors using the same likelihood distribution as that of the posterior with a standard error of 1 (unit).
3. Reference priors that are equal to standardized beta distributions (the standard distribution for binomials) or standardized gamma distributions that are equal to standardized continuous distributions like normal distributions (the standard distributions for normal data).

The mathematics is pretty complex and involves integrating of prior and posterior likelihood distributions and marginalizing out nuisance variables (extraneous variables that cause increase of variability in the statistical model). As an example we will use a hypothesized example with a Poisson frequency distribution. Poisson distributions are convenient because their standard errors (SEs) are the square root of their measured mean λ ($SE = \sqrt{\lambda}$). Poisson distributions are classified among the family of gamma distributions that have an alpha (rate) and a beta (shape) parameter:

$$\text{alpha}(\alpha) = \text{mean} + \left(\text{mean}^2 + 4(\text{standard deviations})^2\right)^2 / 2(\text{standard deviations})^2$$

$$\text{beta}(\beta) = 1 + \text{mean} \times \text{alpha}.$$

As prior here a conjugate prior will be used (as defined above):

the conjugate prior distribution is proportional with $\lambda^{\alpha} e^{-\beta\lambda}$

the posterior distribution $=$ $\lambda^{\alpha+x} e^{-(\beta+1)\lambda}$.

The Bayes factor is computed as the ratio of two likelihood distributions, those of the posterior and the prior:

$$\int \lambda^{\alpha+x} e^{-(\beta+1)\lambda} dx / \int \lambda^{\alpha} e^{-\beta\lambda} dx.$$

The above is only true, if the posterior distribution is proportional to the likelihood distribution multiplied by the prior distribution, where the likelihood distribution is often expressed with the symbols L (θ | data) , meaning the likelihood distribution of an unknown function θ for the data given. Comparable best fit analytic computations can be made for any type of experimental or observational data samples for which a Bayesian analysis is chosen.

1.13   Differences Between Traditional and Bayesian Statistics

With modern Bayesian statistics likelihood distribution rather than probability distribution modeling is applied. It is mostly based on the Cauchy distribution, a member of the family of the alpha distributions, and the distribution that best describes the ratio of two normal distributions or two likelihood distributions. Bayes factors have a Cauchy distribution, and cannot be numerically analyzed with standard Gaussian approximation methods. Fortunately, pretty good numerical results are obtained by integrations that integrate out nuisance variables like those of noninformative priors. With binomial data instead of normal data beta distributions are more adequate, but again integrations are needed for a precise computation of the areas under the curve of the ratios of likelihood distributions. Advantages of the Bayesian approach may include.

1. A better underlying structure model of the H1 and H0 may be provided.
2. Bayesian tests work with 95% credible intervals that are usually somewhat wider and this may reduce the chance of statistical significances with little clinical relevance.
3. Maximal likelihoods of likelihood distributions are not always identical to the mean effect of traditional tests, and this may be fine, because biological likelihoods may better fit biological questions than numerical means of non-representative subgroups do.
4. Bayes uses ratios of likelihood distributions rather than ratios of Gaussian distributions, which are notorious for ill data fit.

5. Bayesian integral computations are very advanced, and, therefore, give optimal precisions of complex functions, and better so than traditional multiple mean calculations of non representative subsamples do.
6. With Bayesian testing type I (otherwise alpha) and II errors (otherwise called beta) need not being taken into account.

The protagonists of Bayesian statistics often argue that the only thing frequentists can do is reject a null hypothesis of no effect or not, and that they are unable to make a sensible statement about the alternative hypothesis H1 (the new treatment has a real effect). This is not entirely true. First of all with a p-value >0.05 the null hypothesis of no effect can not be rejected. It does not necessarily mean that H1 is true, because the study may have been underpowered and with a larger sample size the p-value could as well have been <0.05 and H0 could have been rejected. Second, traditionally the H1 can be assessed with a power assessment. A p = 0.05 means that your type II error of finding a difference where there is one, equals 50%. Next time, we perform the same sized study, we will have a 50% chance of not finding a difference where there is one. If the p-value of your study is much larger than 5%, then the study will increasingly lose power to demonstrate a difference from H0. And this could be interpreted as increasing support for H0 to be true. Along this pattern of p-values from 1 to 0, different levels of support for the H0 and H1 are obtained, just like along the pattern of Bayes factors from ∞ to 0. And so, currently, with traditional testing a power analysis is often performed in combination with a null hypothesis test in order to provide a better underlying structure of the alternative hypothesis H1. This power approach to H1 testing is of course like traditional null hypothesis testing based on Gaussian distributions, and not, like Bayesian procedures, based on likelihood distributions, and, therefore, it does not tell us much which we did not yet know already.

A disadvantage of Bayesian methods may be overfitting. This means that the likelihood distributions are wider than compatible with Gaussian modeling. Bootstraps t-test is based on Monte Carlo resampling from your own data. It is available in SPSS statistical software. In the example given we will compare a bootstraps sampling distribution in SPSS with Bayesian likelihood and traditional Gaussian distributions.

Open the data file entitled "chap6" stored at extras.springer.com in your personal computer mounted with SPSS.

Command:
Analyze....Compare Means....Independent Samples T Test....Dialog Box.... Grouping Variable: enter Group 1 : 1....Group 2: 0....click Bootstrap....click Perform bootstrapping....Number Samples enter 1000....click Continue....click OK.

The bootstrap resampling data is in the output sheets, and provide a 95% confidence interval from
−2.61536 to −0.71752.

The Bayesian and traditional t-test 95% confidence intervals are respectively given:

−2.8098 to −0.6302

−2.73557 to −0.70443

Bootstraps gives the robustest result, but the difference from Bayes or traditional testing does not support much overfitting.

We should add that Bayes factor may sometimes provide a better test statistic than the traditional p-value does (Chap. 5 and 13). However, more often it provides a worse test statistic (Chaps. 6, 7, 8, 12, 13).

1.14   Conclusion

1.14.1   Odds and Probabilities

The odds of having a disease equals the number of patients with the disease divided by the number of patients without the disease (a/b).

disease	yes	no
	a	b

In the above population of (a + b) patients, (a/(a + b)) is the probability of having the disease, while (a/b) is the odds of having a disease. Probabilities are intuitively understood well. They run from 0 to 1. Odds are pretty counterintuitive. Yet they are frequently used in statistics. This is because software programs using odds have a much better performance than those using probabilities. Fortunately, small proportions of probabilities and odds and produce virtually the same, and the interpretation of odds is generally in terms of probability. Odds plays a key role not only in logistic regressions and Cox regressions, but also in traditional Bayes statistical analyses as post-test odds and pre-test odds

1.14.2   Posterior- and Prior-Test Odds

Now, this approach to identifying true positives works fine as long as we have equal chance of disease or not in your study population. However, if the prevalence of disease in your study population is only 20%, then your chance of a positive outcome is much smaller and that of a true positive patients is equally so, despite your likelihood ratio of 16. A 20% prevalence means (with a population of 100) a prior odds of disease of 20/80 = 1/4 instead of 50/50 = 1. Your study outcome will change correspondingly:

$$\text{post   test   odds} = \text{prior   test   odds} \times \text{likelihood   ratio}$$
$$= 1/4 \times 16$$
$$= 4.$$

1.14.3 Traditional Bayes' Theorem

The traditional version of the Bayes' theorem is underneath:

$$\text{Posterior} - \text{test odds} = \text{prior} - \text{test odds} \times \left[\text{sensitivity} / \left(1 - \text{specificity} \right) \right].$$

In a population with both healthy and diseased people the accuracy of a diagnostic test is measured:

1. sensitivity is the fraction of the subjects positive tested divided by all diseased
2. specificity is the fraction of the subjects negative tested divided by all non-diseased.

1.14.4 Modern Bayes

Modern Bayes does not work with normal distributions, but likelihood distributions, that are approximated differently. For continuous data they are pretty tough requiring complex integral computations. For binary data they are more easy to approximate using the binomial distribution. The modern version of Bayes' theorem is below.

$$\text{posterior likelihood distribution} = \text{prior likelihood distribution} \times \left[\text{Bayes factor} \right].$$

1.14.5 Bayes Factor

The traditional Bayes factors is not the AUC of a likelihood distribution curve, but, rather, the ratio of the AUCs of two likelihood distributions. We should add, that the ratio of two odds values, has often been named Bayes factor with traditional Bayesian statistics, but with modern Bayesian statistics, the Bayes factors are mostly based on the ratios of two likelihood distributions. Computations of areas under the curve of nonlinear functions are required.

1.14.6 Achilles Heal of Modern Bayesian Statistics

In the past the non exact intuitive definition of the prior was the Achilles heal. Fortunately, the intuitive prior and the posterior odds have been replaced with more exact likelihood distributions and interpretations based on intervals of uncertainty. However, lacking evidence about priors still exists, and there is a whole battery of tricks to correct for it.

1.14.7 Differences Between Traditional and Bayesian Statistics

1. A better underlying structure of the alternative hypothesis H1 and the null hypothesis H0 may be provided.
2. Bayesian tests work with 95% credible intervals that are usually somewhat wider and this may reduce the chance of statistical significances with little clinical relevance.
3. Maximal likelihoods of likelihood distributions are not always identical to the mean effect of traditional tests, and this may be fine, because biological likelihoods may better fit biological questions than numerical means of non-representative subgroups do.
4. Bayes uses ratios of likelihood distributions rather than ratios of Gaussian distributions, which are notorious for ill data fit.
5. Bayesian integral computations are very advanced, and, therefore, give optimal precisions of complex functions, and better so than traditional multiple mean calculations of non representative subsamples do.
6. With Bayesian testing type I (alpha) and II (beta) errors need not being taken into account.

Suggested Reading[1,2,3]

Statistics applied to clinical studies 5th edition, 2012
Machine learning in medicine a complete overview, 2015
SPSS for starters and 2nd levelers 2nd edition, 2015
Clinical data analysis on a pocket calculator 2nd edition, 2016
Understanding clinical data analysis from published research, 2016
Modern Meta-analysis, 2017
Regression Analysis in Clinical Research, 2018

---

[1] To readers requesting more background, theoretical and mathematical information of computations given, several textbooks complementary to the current production and written by the same authors are available.

[2] All of them have been written by the same authors, and they have been edited by Springer Heidelberg Germany.

[3] The recent FDA's Guidance for the use of Bayesian statistics in medical device clinical trials (February 2010) is a helpful stepwise learning text from evidence as it accumulates and particularly written for novices in the field.

Chapter 2
Traditional Bayes: Diagnostic Testing, Genetic Data Analyses, Bayes and Drug Trials

2.1 Background

In clinical research where the base rate for a disease is very low and the diagnostic test is far from perfect, there will be a pretty high probability of a positive result that is false positive. In order to determine the probability of a positive test being accurate, you need to account the following.

1. the base rate that have the disease irrespective of the test results.
2. the sensitivity of your test, which is the proportion of true positive patients to be expected.
3. the specificity of your test, which is the proportion of true negative patients to be expected.

The posterior odds is the ratio of true positive and true negative patients in your study. The prior odds is the same ratio but obtained from historic data. The underneath equation can be used to compute the posterior odds.

$$\text{Prior test odds} \times \text{Bayes factor} = \text{posterior test odds}.$$

Thomas Bayes from London UK, 1760, was English clergyman and mathematician/statistician who developed an interesting probability theory helpful to analyze qualitative diagnostic tests. This theory was later called Bayes' theorem. The Bayes factor can be briefly rewritten as.

$$\text{Bayes factor} = \left[\text{sensitivity} / \left(1 - \text{specificity}\right) \right].$$

The Bayes' theorem has been traditionally used for three main purposes:

1. diagnostic testing,
2. genetic data analyses,
3. finding the probability in drug trials that a new drug will really work.

© Springer International Publishing AG, part of Springer Nature 2018
T. J. Cleophas, A. H. Zwinderman, *Modern Bayesian Statistics in Clinical Research*,
https://doi.org/10.1007/978-3-319-92747-3_2

2.2   Diagnostic Testing

Generally, with quantitative diagnostic tests accuracy is assessed with complex linear regression methods like Passing Bablok regressions (Statistics applied to clinical studies 5th edition, pp 551–553, Springer Heidelberg Germany, 2012, from the same authors). However, for simplicity the results can also be reported in the form of two normal distributions with healthy and diseased and an arbitrary cut-off between the two. The underneath graph shows the summary of a random sample of people at risk of a disease with test results on the x-axis and probability density on the y-axis. The summary is in the form of two Gaussian-like areas under the curve. *Left curve* are healthy subjects, *right curve* are diseased. The graph is comparable to the graph of two Gaussians shown in Chap. 1, but there is also a difference. The area under the curve of the right curve is much smaller than that of the left curve. This would mean that the number of diseased is much smaller than the numbers of healthy subjects.

TP = true positives = area under the small curve without the grey triangle
FP = false positives = surface of black triangle
TN = true negatives = area under the large curve without the black triangle
FN = false negatives = surface of grey triangle.

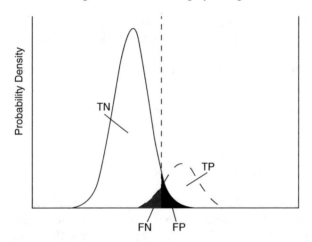

1. *Rare Disease*

    Rare diseases may have a prevalence of 4/10,000 = 40/100,000 at best.

    If such a disease can be diagnosed with a test, and this test has a sensitivity of 82%, specificity of 94%, then the ratio of TP/ (TP + FN) and TN/(TN + FP) = sensitivity/(1 − specificity) = 0.82/(1 − 0.94) = 13.6667. This term gives the probability of obtaining a positive test in a patient without the disease as compared to the probability of obtaining a positive test in patients without the disease, and is often called likelihood ratio of a positive test in negative patients, or, simply, likelihood ratio, or Bayes factor.

    Suppose we have 100,000 random patients: 40 of them will have the disease.

Disease	Yes	No	Together
Positive test	0.82 × 40 = 32.8	0.06 × 99,960 = 5997.6	6030.4
negative test	0.18 × 40 = 7.2	0.94 × 99,960 = 93962.4	93969.6
together	40	99,960	100,000

After *screening* 100,000 patients we will find 32.8 diseased patients and this is a proportion of 32.8/6030.4 = 0.005439 of all patients with positive tests. This means, that 0.54% of all positive patients will have the disease.

An slightly different way to find this result is the Bayes equation.

$$\text{Prior test odds} \times \text{Bayes factor}$$
$$= \text{posterior test odds.}$$

$$(40 / 99960) \times \text{Bayes factor}$$
$$= \text{posterior test odds.}$$

$$\text{Bayes factor} = \text{sensitivity} / (1 - \text{specificity})$$
$$= 0.82 / (1 - 0.94)$$
$$= 13.6667.$$

$$\text{Posterior test odds}$$
$$= (40 / 99960) \times 13.6667$$
$$= 0.00547$$

The posterior test odds equals again the patients with a positive test and diseased as compared to those with a positive test and no disease. This is an odds term, and in order to find the proportion of diseased patients we need to transform the odds into the chance or probability.Probability = 1/(1 + 1/odds) = 1/ (1 + 1/0.00547) = 0.005439.This means, that only 0.54% of all positive patients will have the disease. The chance of 0.54 % is very small, but, as a first screening, it may do.

2. *More Common Disease*
   More common diseases may have a prevalence of 10% = 100/1000. If, like in the above section, such a disease can be diagnosed with a sensitivity of 82%, specificity of 94%, then the ratio sensitivity/(1 − specificity) = 0.82/ (1 − 0.94) = 13.6667. The underneath Bayesian equation is used for finding the proportion of positive patients that are really diseased.

$$\text{Prior test odds} \times \text{Bayes factor}$$
$$= \text{posterior test odds.}$$

$$(100 / 900) \times \text{Bayes factor}$$
$$= \text{posterior test odds.}$$

$$\text{Bayes factor} = \text{sensitivity} / (1 - \text{specificity})$$
$$= 0.82 / (1 - 0.94)$$
$$= 13.6667.$$

Posterior test odds
$$= (100 / 900) \times 13.6667$$
$$= 1.519$$

The posterior test odds equals again the patients with a positive test and diseased as compared to those with a positive test and no disease. This is an odds term, and in order to find the proportion of diseased patients we need to transform the odds into the chance or probability.

Probability = 1/(1 + 1/odds) = 1/(1 + 1/1.519) = 0.603.

This means, that 60.3% of all positive patients will have the disease. The chance of 60.3% is pretty good, but we still have many false positives.

3. *Common Disease*

Common diseases may have a prevalence of 30% = 300/1000. If, like in the above section, such a disease can again be diagnosed with a sensitivity of 82%, specificity of 94%, then the ratio sensitivity/(1 − specificity) = 0.82/(1 − 0.94) = 13.6667. The underneath Bayesian equation is used for finding the proportion of positive patients that are really diseased.

$$\text{Prior test odds} \times \text{Bayes factor}$$
$$= \text{posterior test odds.}$$

$$(300 / 700) \times \text{Bayes factor}$$
$$= \text{posterior test odds.}$$

$$\text{Bayes factor} = \text{sensitivity} / (1 - \text{specificity})$$
$$= 0.82 / (1 - 0.94)$$
$$= 13.6667.$$

Posterior test odds
$$= (300 / 700) \times 13.6667$$
$$= 5.857$$

The posterior test odds equals again the patients with a positive test and diseased as compared to those with a positive test and no disease. This is an odds term, and in order to find the proportion of diseased patients we need to transform the odds into the chance or probability.

Probability = 1/(1 + 1/odds) = 1/(1 + 1/5.857) = 0.854.

This means, that 85.4% of all positive patients will have the disease. The chance of 85.4 % is good, and we will have only 14.6% false positives.

4. *Very common disease like a genetic disease with 50% gene carrier ship*
Very common diseases may have a prevalence of 50% = 500/1000. If, like in the above section, such a disease can again be diagnosed with a sensitivity of 82%, specificity of 94%, then the ratio sensitivity/(1 − specificity) = 0.82/(1 − 0.94) = 13.6667. The underneath Bayesian equation is used for finding the proportion of positive patients that are really diseased.

$$\text{Prior test odds} \times \text{Bayes factor}$$
$$= \text{posterior test odds.}$$

$$(500/500) \times \text{Bayes factor}$$
$$= \text{posterior test odds.}$$

$$\text{Bayes factor} = \text{sensitivity} / (1 - \text{specificity})$$
$$= 0.82 / (1 - 0.94)$$
$$= 13.6667.$$

$$\text{Posterior test odds}$$
$$= (500/500) \times 13.6667$$
$$= 13.6667$$

The posterior test odds equals again the patients with a positive test and diseased as compared to those with a positive test and no disease. This is an odds term, and in order to find the proportion of diseased patients we need to transform the odds into the chance or probability.

Probability = 1/(1 + 1/odds) = 1/(1 + 1/13.6667) = 0.932.

This means, that 93.2% of all positive patients will have the disease. The chance of 93.2% is excellent, and we will have only 6.8% false positives.

5. *Example of disease with 75% prevalence in a population*
Epidemic diseases may have a prevalence of 75% = 750/1000. If, like in the above section, such a disease can again be diagnosed with a sensitivity of 82%, specificity of 94%, then the ratio sensitivity/(1 − specificity) = 0.82/(1 − 0.94) = 13.6667. The underneath Bayesian equation is used for finding the proportion of positive patients that are really diseased.

$$\text{Prior test odds} \times \text{Bayes factor}$$
$$= \text{posterior test odds.}$$

$$(750/250) \times \text{Bayes factor}$$
$$= \text{posterior test odds.}$$

$$\text{Bayes factor} = \text{sensitivity} / (1 - \text{specificity})$$
$$= 0.82 / (1 - 0.94)$$
$$= 13.6667.$$

Posterior test odds

$$= (750 / 250) \times 13.6667$$
$$= 41.0001$$

The posterior test odds equals again the patients with a positive test and diseased as compared to those with a positive test and no disease. This is an odds term, and in order to find the proportion of diseased patients we need to transform the odds into the chance or probability.

Probability = 1/(1 + 1/odds) = 1/(1 + 1/41.0001) = 0.976.

This means, that 97.6% of all positive patients will have the disease. The chance of 97.6 % is excellent, and we will have only 2.4% false positives.

The above examples show how the Bayes factor can conveniently used to assess the chance of true positive tests out of a sample of positive tests. The larger the prior test odds the better chance is given. Finding true positives in a population with lots of false positives is a useful purpose for traditional Bayesian statistics. Other traditional Bayesian statistics are analyses of genetic data and the analysis of clinical trial data with power assessed a priori.

2.3   Analysis of Genetic Data

Some basic terms used with genetic data analysis are given.

Bayes' Theorem	Posterior odds = likelihood ratio x prior odds
	This approach is required for making predictions from genetic data. Although the general concept of including prior evidence in the statistical analysis of clinical trial data is appealing, this concept should not be applied in usual null-hypothesis testing, because we would have to violate the main assumption of null-hypothesis testing that H0 and H1 have the same frequency distribution.
Posterior odds	Prior odds adjusted for likelihood ratio.
Prior odds	Prior probability of being a carrier/prior probability of being no carrier.
Likelihood ratio	Probability for carriers of having healthy offspring/probability for non-carrier of having healthy offspring.
Genetic linkage	When two genes or DNA sequences are located near each other on the same chromosome, they are linked. When they are not close, crossing over occurs frequently. However, when they are close they tend to be inherited together. Genetic linkage is useful in genetic diagnosis and mapping because once you know that the disease gene is linked to a particular DNA sequence that is close, the latter can be used as a marker to identify the disease gene indirectly. Bayes' Theorem can be used to combine experimental data with prior linkage probabilities as established.

Bayes' Theorem is an important approach for the analysis of genetic data. An example will be given. Based on historical data the chance for girls in a particular family of being carrier for the hemophilia A gene is 50%. Those who are carrier will have a chance of $\frac{1}{2} \times \frac{1}{2} = \frac{1}{4} = 25\%$ that two sons are healthy. Those who are no carriers will have a 100% chance of two healthy sons. This would mean that a girl from this population who had two healthy sons is 500/125 = 4 times more likely to be no carrier than to be carrier. In terms of Bayes' Theorem:

posterior odds = prior odds x likelihood ratio.	
prior probability of being carrier = 50%	
prior odds = 50:50 = 1.0	
likelihood ratio	= probability for carrier of having two healthy sons/probability for non-carrier of having two healthy sons
	= 25%/100%
	= 0.25 posterior odds
	= 1.0 times 0.25
	= 25% or 1 in 4.

If you saw many girls from this family you would see one carrier for every four non-carriers.

mothers with two sons who are:	carrier	no carrier
	n = 500	n = 500
two sons healthy	n = 125	n = 500
two sons not healthy	n = 375	n = 0.

2.4   Bayes and Drug Trials

Motulsky in Intuitive Statistics pp 129–152 (Oxford University Press 1995) gave an interesting example of including in drug trials prior probability estimates that a drug will work. They are, then, applied for assessing the posterior odds of a positive trial. Nowadays trials are often sample-sized such that they will produce both a 5% chance of a false positive result and 20% chance of a false negative result, otherwise called 5% type I and 20% type II error.

With only a 1% prior probability (prob) of successful treatment the posterior odds of success is computed.

	Prob that drug will work	will not work	total
Positive trial	0.008	0.05	0.058
negative trial	0.002	0.94	0.942
prior prob	0.01	0.99	1.0

posterior odds of success	= 0.008/0.05,
posterior probability of success	= 0.008/0.058
	= 0.138
	= 13.8%.

With a 10% prior probability of successful treatment the posterior odds of success is computed.

	Prob that drug will work	will not work	total
Positive trial	0.08	0.045	0.125
negative trial	0.02	0.855	0.875
prior prob	0.10	0.90	1.0

posterior odds of success	= 0.08/0.045,
posterior probability of success	= 0.08/0.125
	= 0.64
	= 64%.

With a 80% prior probability of successful treatment the posterior odds of success is computed.

	Prob that drug will work	will not work	total
Positive trial	0.64	0.01	0.65
negative trial	0.16	0.19	0.35
prior prob	0.8	0.2	1.0

posterior odds of success	= 0.64/0.01,
posterior probability of success	= 0.64/0.65
	= 98.5%.

Obviously, the higher the prior probability, the better posterior probability of success. We should add that prior probability is usually more a subjective feeling than a really objectively measured probability. Unlike with genetic linkage prior information is usually far from exact.

With traditional statistical testing we have no information about prior probabilities, and the probability of a successful treatment is dependent only on the magnitudes of the type I and II errors. If the type II error (= beta) can be assumed to be 20% (power is 80%), and the type I error (= alpha) 5%, then the chance of real efficacy equals

$$80/(80+5) = 80/85 = 94.1\%.$$

This is, because the chance of finding a significant test equals (1 − beta + alpha) = (80 + 5)%, while 5% is the type I error of finding an effect where there is none.

It would mean that we have $100 - 94.1 = 5.9\%$ chance of a real lack of efficacy.

In summary.

Without prior knowledge, we will have 94.1% chance that the drug is really efficacious if a p-value of 0.05 is observed.
With prior knowledge of 1% this chance reduces to only 13.8%.
With prior knowledge of 10% this chance reduces to only 64%.
With prior knowledge of 80% this chance increases to 98.5%.

In conclusion with Bayes and prior knowledge of low chances of efficacy, the chance that the drug is really efficacious is *smaller* than that with traditional testing. However, with prior knowledge of high chances of efficacy, the chance that the drug is really efficacious is *larger* than that with traditional testing. Obviously, Bayes testing is sometimes somewhat counterintuitive, and does not always produce results that are directly in correspondence with the traditional methods. Careful computations are, therefore, required.

2.5 Conclusion

This chapter has reviewed three (3) methodologies where traditional Bayesian statistics is applied. Diagnostic testing (first) and implying prior probability in drug trials (second) are rather subjective, while so far the only more exact application of Bayesian statistics is genetic data analysis (third). In the next chapters we will address modern Bayesian statistics that instead of post and prior tests odds makes use of post and prior tests likelihood distributions. With modern Bayesian statistics the invariant Bayes factor consistent of the likelihood ratio of a prior and posterior odds has been replaced with a Bayes factor consistent of two likelihood *distributions*. They have, in addition to maximal likelihoods, distributions of likelihoods. As a consequence, the novel BFs have intervals with different levels of support of the presence of some outcome. All of this is pretty new, but advantages, although so far unproven, have been mentioned. Bayesian tests work with 95% credible intervals that are usually somewhat wider than the traditional 95% confidence intervals, and this is fine, because it may reduce the chance of statistical significances with little clinical relevance. Also maximal likelihoods of likelihood distributions are not always identical to the mean effect of traditional tests, and this may be so, because biological likelihoods better fit biological questions than numerical means do. In addition, Bayesian not only uses likelihood distributions but also ratios of likelihood distributions (Cauchy distributions) rather than ratios of Gaussian distributions, the latter of which are notorious for ill data fit. Fourth, Bayesian integral computations are very advanced, and, therefore, give optimal precisions of complex functions, and better so than traditional multiple mean calculations of non representative subsamples do. Fifth, with modern Bayesian statistics type I and II errors need not being taken into account. Obviously, all of this sounds promising, and in the past few years many scientists including econo-, socio-, psychometricians are rather satisfied with the result patterns of modern Bayesian data analyses.

From now on in this edition prior and posterior likelihood distributions instead of prior and posterior odds will be applied, and for convenience they will be briefly named priors and posteriors.

Suggested Reading[1,2]

Statistics applied to clinical studies 5th edition, 2012
Machine learning in medicine a complete overview, 2015
SPSS for starters and 2nd levelers 2nd edition, 2015
Clinical data analysis on a pocket calculator 2nd edition, 2016
Understanding clinical data analysis from published research, 2016
Modern Meta-analysis, 2017
Regression Analysis in Clinical Research, 2018

---

[1] To readers requesting more background, theoretical and mathematical information of computations given, several textbooks complementary to the current production and written by the same authors are available.

[2] All of them have been written by the same authors and have been edited by Springer Heidelberg Germany.

Chapter 3
Bayesian Tests for One Sample Continuous Data

3.1 Background

In studies with one sample continuous data Xa single outcome per patient is usually compared to zero. They may be analyzed with the one sample t-test, that is, if data can be assumed to follow a Gaussian-like pattern. The test assesses whether the mean outcome and its 95% confidence interval (the alternative hypothesis H1) is significantly different from the value zero and the same 95% confidence interval (the null hypothesis H0). Instead of t-test also a Bayesian one sample normal test is possible. It assesses the magnitude of the Bayes factor (BF). A BF smaller than "one" supports the above alternative hypothesis (H1), while a BF larger than "one" supports the above null hypothesis (H0). The BF is computed as the ratio of two likelihood distributions, that of the posterior and the prior likelihood distribution. The first is modeled from the mean and standard deviation of the measured data, the second can be modeled from the variance of the posterior data but a uniform prior with a likelihood of "one" in the same interval as that of the posterior is pretty much OK as well. The computation of the BF requires integrations for accuracy purposes. But, then, it can be used as a statistical index to pretty precisely quantify the amount of support in favor H1 and H0. Advantages of the Bayesian approach may include:

1. A better underlying structure model of both the alternative and null hypothesis may be provided.
2. Maximal likelihoods of likelihood distributions are not always identical to the mean effect of traditional tests, and this may be fine, because biological likelihoods may better fit biological questions than numerical means of non-representative subgroups do.

However, in spite of this, nobody knows for sure why likelihood distributions may better than normal distributions estimate uncertainties in statistical test results. So, why not use both of them for analyzing the same data example. The current chapter will show and compare the results of traditional one sample t-tests and Bayesian one sample t-tests.

© Springer International Publishing AG, part of Springer Nature 2018
T. J. Cleophas, A. H. Zwinderman, *Modern Bayesian Statistics in Clinical Research*,
https://doi.org/10.1007/978-3-319-92747-3_3

3.2 Example

In a 10 patient hypertension study the primary scientific question was: is the observed reduction of mean blood pressure after treatment larger than zero reduction. For convenience the data file is in extras.springer.com, and is entitled "chap3".

Var

3,00
4,00
-1,00
3,00
2,00
-2,00
4,00
3,00
-1,00
2,00

Var = decrease of mean blood pressure after treatment (mmHg) (Var = variable)

3.3 Traditional One-Sample T-Test

Start by opening the data file in your computer mounted with SPSS version 25 with the advanced statistics module included.

Command:
Analyze....Compare Means....One Sample T-Test....Test Variable: enter Var 00001....click OK.

In the output the underneath table is given.

One-sample test

	Test value = 0				95% Confidence interval of the difference	
	t	df	Sig. (2-tailed)	Mean difference	Lower	Upper
VAR00001	2,429	9	,038	1,70000	,1165	3,2835

The above table shows that the t-value equals 2.429, which means that with $(10 - 1) = 9$ degrees of freedom a significant effect is obtained with $p = 0.038$.

The reduction of mean blood pressure has an average value of 1.7 mmHg, and this average reduction is significantly larger than a reduction of 0 mmHg. The null hypothesis of a t-value not significantly different from zero is rejected at p = 0.038.

3.4 Bayesian One-Sample T-Test

We think that the null hypothesis may be rejected erroneously due to a type I error, and will perform a Bayesian analysis to find additional evidence.

Command:
Bayesian Statistics....One Sample Normal....Test Variable: enter Var 00001....Bayesian Analysis: mark Use Both Methods....click Criteria: Credible interval percentage %: 95....click Continue....mark Variance....Prior Distribution: Diffuse....click Continue....click OK.

The underneath tables and graphs are in the output sheets. The Bayes factor is estimated from the ratio of a prior and posterior likelihood distribution. The posterior distribution is based on the means of the measured values. Credible intervals are computed from its likelihood distribution assuming here a normal distribution. The prior likelihood distribution is not given in the current example. Yet, a Bayes factor is computed as well as the mode, mean, and 95% credible interval of the posterior likelihood distribution.

Bayes factor for one-sample T test

	N	Mean	Std. deviation	Std. error mean	Bayes factor[a]	t	df	Sig. (2-tailed)
Mean blood pressure reduction	10	1,7000	2,21359	,70000	,506	2,429	9	,038

[a]Bayes factor, Null versus alternative hypothesis

Posterior distribution characterization for one-sample mean

	N	Posterior Mean	Posterior Mean	Variance	95% Credible interval Lower bound	95% Credible interval Upper bound
Mean blood pressure reduction	10	1,7000	1,7000	,882	−,1769	3,5769

Prior on variance: diffuse. Prior on mean: diffuse

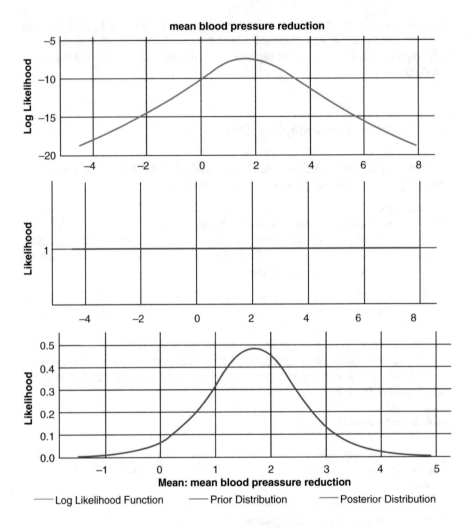

Particularly the above second and third graph are of interest. The second graph shows a prior likelihood distribution, based on the variance of the posterior. It is the simplest possible prior, otherwise called non-informative uniform prior with a function of f x = 1. This is not a nonsense solution for lack of information in the data, and it even makes a lot of sense, because it has the form that can be integrated out in the analysis. The graph shows that in the interval between a mean blood pressure reduction between −1 and 5, its area under the curve can be easily roughly estimated (see Chap. 1), but integration is more accurate. The third graph gives the posterior likelihood distribution in the form of a normal distribution with 1.700 as mode and mean.

The computed Bayes factor of 0.506 supports that the null hypothesis of no difference from zero blood pressure reduction has rightly been be rejected in the above one sample t-test. However, the level of evidence (anecdotal support for the alternative hypothesis, H1, see underneath table given by SPSS) is not strong. Also the computed credible interval is wider than it is for the traditional one sample t-test. The credible intervals are between -0.1769 and 3.5769 as compared to 0.1165–3.2835 for the 95% confidence intervals of the traditional one sample t-test.

Bayes factor	Evidence category	Bayes factor	Evidence category	Bayes factor	Evidence category
>100	Extreme evidence for H0	1–3	Anecdotal evidence for H0	1/30 to 1/10	Strong evidence for H1
30–100	Very strong evidence for H0	1	No evidence	1/100 to 1/30	Very strong evidence for H1
10–30	Strong evidence for H0	1/3 to 1	Anecdotal evidence for H1	1/100	Extreme evidence for H1
3–10	Moderate evidence for H0	1/10 to 1/3	Moderate evidence for H1		

The above table is helpful for interpretation of the measured Bayes factors of your data. A very small Bayes factor corresponds to a very small p-value. The underneath red diagonal is helpful too, Bayes factor values above one support the rejection of the alternative hypothesis, H1. Values below 1 support the rejection of the null hypothesis, H0.

Reject H1

Bayes Factor	Evidence Category	Bayes Factor	Evidence Category	Bayes Factor	Evidence Category
>100	Extreme Evidence for H0	1-3	Anecdotal Evidence for H0	1/30-1/10	Strong Evidence for H1
30-100	Very Strong Evidence for H0	1	No Evidence	1/100-1/30	Very Strong Evidence for H1
10-30	Strong Evidence for H0	1/3-1	Anecdotal Evidence for H1	1/100	Extreme Evidence for H1
3-10	Moderate Evidence for H0	1/10-1/3	Moderate Evidence for H1		

Reject H0

3.5 Conclusion

This chapter assesses the Bayesian one sample t-test. The results are pretty similar to those of the traditional one sample t-test. The Bayesian t-test provides less precision in support of the alternative hypothesis than the traditional t-test does, but considering the small sample the precision of the traditional test may indeed be somewhat overstated.

With modern Bayesian statistics likelihood distributions rather than probability distribution are modeled. The ratios of the posterior and prior likelihood distributions are supposedly based on the Cauchy distribution, a member of the family of the alpha distributions, and they are the distribution that best describes the ratio of two normal distributions as well as two likelihood distributions. Bayes factors having Cauchy distribution, cannot be numerically analyzed with standard Gaussian approximation methods. Fortunately, pretty good numerical results are obtained by integrations that integrate out nuisance variables like the variables of noninformative priors or lacking priors. With binomial data instead of normal distributions beta distributions are more adequate, but integrations are again needed. An example is given in the next chapter.

Advantages of the Bayesian approach may include.

1. A better underlying structure of the H1 and H0 may be provided.
2. Bayesian tests work with 95% credible intervals that are usually somewhat wider and this may reduce the chance of statistical significances with little clinical relevance.
3. Maximal likelihoods of likelihood distributions are not always identical to the mean effect of traditional tests, and this may be fine, because biological likelihoods may better fit biological questions than numerical means of non-representative subgroups do.
4. Bayes uses ratios of likelihood distributions rather than ratios of Gaussian distributions, which are notorious for ill data fit.
5. Bayesian integral computations are very advanced, and, therefore, give optimal precisions of complex functions, and better so than traditional multiple mean calculations of non representative subsamples do.
6. With Bayesian testing type I and II errors need not being taken into account.

A disadvantage of Bayesian methods may be overfitting. This means that the likelihood distributions may be wider than compatible with Gaussian modeling. Bootstraps t-test is based on Monte Carlo resampling from your own data. It is available in SPSS statistical software. In the example given we will compare a bootstraps sampling distribution in SPSS with Bayesian likelihood and traditional Gaussian distributions. For that purpose we will use again the same data file and the same statistical software. Open again the data file entitled "chap3" stored at extras.springer.com in your personal computer mounted with SPSS.

Command:
Analyze....Compare Means....One Sample T-Test....Test Variable: enter Var 00001....click Bootstrap....click Perform bootstrapping....Number Samples enter 1000....click Continue....click OK.

The bootstrap resampling model is in the output sheets. It provides a 95% confidence interval between 0.400 and 2.900.

The Bayesian and traditional t-test 95% confidence intervals are given above.

1. Gaussian 95% confidence interval 0.1165–3.2835
2. Bootstrap 95% confidence interval 0.4000 and 2.9000
3. Bayesian 95% credible interval −0.1769 and 3.5769.

Obviously, the Gaussian confidence interval is wider than bootstrap confidence interval, while the Bayesian credible interval is the widest. Assuming that the bootstraps model is entirely without overfitting, some degree of overfitting, both of the Gaussian, and, even more, of the Bayesian model can not be ruled out.

The Bayes factor (BF) in this chapter's example of 0.506 would suggest that the Bayesian one sample t-test model provides a slightly better sensitivity of testing than the traditional one sample continuous data t-test model did.

On a continuous line of Bayes factors from 1.0 to 0.0, our Bayes factor is in the middle.

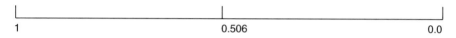

1   0.506   0.0

On a continuous line of p-values from 0.05 to 0.0 our p-value is skewed to the left end side.

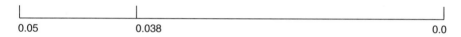

0.05   0.038   0.0

The BF of 0.506 is closer to 0.0 (or very small), than a p-value of 0.038 is. The BF provides a better statistic here than does the p-value.

Suggested Reading[1,2]

Statistics applied to clinical studies 5th edition, 2012
Machine learning in medicine a complete overview, 2015
SPSS for starters and 2nd levelers 2nd edition, 2015
Clinical data analysis on a pocket calculator 2nd edition, 2016
Understanding clinical data analysis from published research, 2016
Regression Analysis in Clinical Research, 2018

---

[1] To readers requesting more background, theoretical and mathematical information of computations given, several textbooks complementary to the current production and written by the same authors are available.

[2] All of them have been written by the same authors, and have been edited by Springer Heidelberg Germany.

Chapter 4
Bayesian Tests for One Sample Binary Data

4.1 Background

In studies with one sample of binomial data (yes no data) the z-test is pretty much traditionally used for analysis. It tests whether the ratio of the mean and its standard error is larger than 1.96. The alternative hypothesis (H1) is defined as the mean proportion ± twice its standard error (otherwise called its 95% confidence interval) and the null hypothesis (H0) as a proportion of being zero ± twice the same standard error. Instead of z-test also a Bayesian one sample binomial test is possible. It assesses the magnitude of the Bayes factor (BF). A BF smaller than "one" supports the above alternative hypothesis (H1), while a BF larger than "one" supports the above null hypothesis (H0). The BF is computed as the ratio of two likelihood distributions, that of the posterior and the prior likelihood distribution. The first is modeled from the mean proportion and standard error of the measured data, the second can be modeled from a conjugate pattern of the posterior (this is the same pattern) or from a reference prior using a standard beta distribution with 0.5 as mean responder and an interval between 0 and 1. The computation of the BF requires integrations for accuracy purposes. But, then, it can be used as a statistical index to pretty precisely quantify the amount of support in favor H1 and H0. Advantages of the Bayesian approach may include.

1. A better underlying structure model of the H1 and H0 may be provided.
2. Maximal likelihoods of likelihood distributions are not always identical to the mean effect of traditional tests, and this may be fine, because biological likelihoods may better fit biological questions than numerical means of non-representative subgroups do.

However, in spite of this, nobody knows for sure why likelihood distributions may better than normal distributions estimate uncertainties in statistical test results. So, why not use both of them for analyzing the same data example. The current chapter will show and compare the results of traditional binomial and Bayesian binomial tests.

© Springer International Publishing AG, part of Springer Nature 2018
T. J. Cleophas, A. H. Zwinderman, *Modern Bayesian Statistics in Clinical Research*,
https://doi.org/10.1007/978-3-319-92747-3_4

4.2   Example

A hypertension study of 55 patients has as primary scientific question: is the number of patients who respond significantly larger than a number of 0. For convenience the data file is in extras.springer.com and is entitled "chap4".

Var 1
,00
,00
,00
,00
,00
,00
,00
,00
,00
,00
,00
,00
,00
,00
,00
,00
,00
,00
,00
,00
,00
,00
,00
,00
,00
,00
,00
,00
,00
,00
,00
,00
,00
,00
,00
1,00
1,00

Var 1
1,00
1,00
1,00
1,00
1,00
1,00
1,00
1,00
1,00
1,00
1,00
1,00
1,00
1,00
1,00
1,00
1,00
1,00

Var 1 = responder to antihypertensive drug or not (1 or 0) (Var = variable)

4.3   Traditional Analysis of Binary Data with the Z-Test

Start by opening the data file in your computer mounted with SPSS statistical software version 25 with the module advanced statistics included.

Command:
Analyze....Descriptive Statistics....Descriptives....Variable(s): enter Var 00001....
    Options: mark mean, sum, SE mean....click Continue....click OK.

Descriptive statistics

	N	Sum	Mean	
	Statistic	Statistic	Statistic	Std. error
afdeling	55	20,00	,3636	,06546
Valid N (listwise)	55			

The z-value as obtained equals 0.3636/0.06546 = 5.5545. This z-value is much larger than 1.96, and, therefore, the null hypothesis of no difference from a proportion of 0 can be rejected with p < 0.001. This proportion of 20/55 is significantly different from 0. The null hypothesis of no difference from zero is rejected.

4.4   Analysis: Bayesian Statistics One Sample Binomial

We think that the null hypothesis may have been rejected erroneously and that due to the small data sample size type I errors cannot be ruled out. A Bayesian analysis may provide additional evidence.

Command:
Bayesian Statistics....One Sample Binomial....Test Variable: enter responder (VAR 00001)....Bayesian Analysis: mark Use Both Methods....click Criteria: Credible interval percentage %: 95....click Continue....mark Priors: Alternate Prior Shape: enter 2....Alternate Prior Scale: enter 2....click Continue....click OK.

The underneath tables and graphs are in the output sheets. The Bayes factor (BF) is estimated from the ratio of the likelihood distribution of the proportional difference from zero and the likelihood distribution of a standard beta distribution with 0.5 as max and with an interval from 0 to 1 (called a reference prior). The posterior distribution is based on the actual proportion of responders as measured. Credible intervals are computed from its likelihood distribution assuming a binomial distribution from the family of beta distributions. Defaults for shape and scales were entered.

Bayes-factor for binomial proportion test

		Observed			
	Success category	N	Successes	Proportion	Bayes factor
Responder	=1,00	55	20	,364	1,000

Bayes factor. Null versus alternative hypothesis

Posterior distribution characterization for binomial inference[a]

	Posterior			95% Credible interval	
	Mode	Mean	Var.	Lower bound	Upper bound
Responder	,368	,373	,004	,255	,499

[a]Prior on Binomial proportion: Beta(2,2)

The BF and the 95% credible intervals of the posterior likelihood distribution are given in the above output tables. Also in the output sheets are the underneath three graphs.

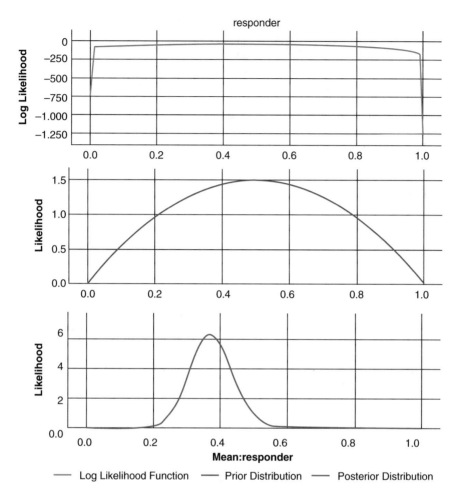

— Log Likelihood Function   — Prior Distribution   — Posterior Distribution

Particularly the above second and third graph are of interest. The second graph
shows a prior likelihood distribution based on the standard beta distribution curve
with 0.5 as mean responder and an interval between 0 and 1. The third graph gives
the posterior likelihood distribution is in the form of a skewed likelihood distribution with 0.368 as mode and 0.373 as mean. The computed Bayes factor (BF) of
1.000 shows that the traditional alternative hypothesis is on the verge of being supported. However, the level of evidence (only anecdotal support for the alternative
hypothesis, H1, is not strong. See underneath table given by SPSS. Also the computed credible interval is wider than it is for the traditional one sample t-test (or
rather called here one sample z-test). The 95% credible interval between 0.256 and
0.499 is a bit wider than the 95% confidence interval from SPSS's Descriptives
table (not given) for the 95% confidence interval of the z-test (0.2327 and 0.4945).
With a BF of 1.000 obviously less support in favor of the alternative hypothesis is
given as compared to that of the above z-test.

Bayes factor	Evidence category	Bayes factor	Evidence category	Bayes factor	Evidence category
>100	Extreme evidence for H0	1–3	Anecdotal evidence for H0	1/30 to 1/10	Strong evidence for H1
30–100	Very strong evidence for H0	1	No evidence	1/100 to1/30	Very strong evidence for H1
10–30	Strong evidence for H0	1/3 to 1	Anecdotal evidence for H1	1/100	Extreme evidence for H1
3–10	Moderate evidence for H0	1/10 to 1/3	Moderate evidence for H1		

The table is helpful for interpretation of the measured BFs of your data. Generally they pretty much look like traditional statistics: a very small Bayes factor corresponds to a very small p-value. The underneath red diagonal is helpful too, Bayes factor values above-one support the rejection of the traditional alternative hypothesis, H1. Values below-one support the rejection of the null hypothesis, H0.

Reject H1

Bayes Factor	Evidence Category	Bayes Factor	Evidence Category	Bayes Factor	Evidence Category
>100	Extreme Evidence for H0	1-3	Anecdotal Evidence for H0	1/30-1/10	Strong Evidence for H1
30-100	Very Strong Evidence for H0	1	No Evidence	1/100-1/30	Very Strong Evidence for H1
10-30	Strong Evidence for H0	1/3-1	Anecdotal Evidence for H1	1/100	Extreme Evidence for H1
3-10	Moderate Evidence for H0	1/10/-1/3	Moderate Evidence for H1		

Reject H0

4.5   Conclusion

This chapter assesses the Bayesian one sample test for binary data. The results are pretty similar to those of the traditional z-test for the purpose. The Bayesian t-test provides less precision in support of the alternative hypothesis than the traditional t-test does. However, considering the small data in the example the traditional z-test may have somewhat overstated certainty, and the Bayesian test may, therefore, be somewhat more realistic.

Advantages of the Bayesian approach may include.

1. A better underlying structure of the H1 and H0 may be provided.
2. Bayesian tests work with 95% credible intervals that are usually somewhat wider and this may reduce the chance of statistical significances with little clinical relevance.
3. Maximal likelihoods of likelihood distributions are not always identical to the mean effect of traditional tests, and this may be fine, because biological likelihoods may better fit biological questions than numerical means of non-representative subgroups do.
4. Bayes uses ratios of likelihood distributions rather than ratios of Gaussian distributions, which are notorious for ill data fit.
5. Bayesian integral computations are very advanced, and, therefore, give optimal precisions of complex functions, and better so than traditional multiple mean calculations of non representative subsamples do.
6. With Bayesian testing type I and II errors need not being taken into account.

The Bayes factor (BF) in this chapter's example of 1.0 suggests that the Bayesian test for one sample binary data provides a very poor sensitivity of testing as compared to that of the p-value of 0.001 of the traditional one sample binary data test.

On a continuous line of BFs from 1.0 to 0.0, our BF is very much skewed to the left end side.

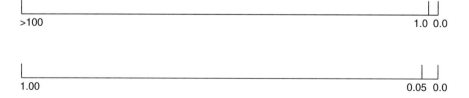

1.0   0.0

On a continuous line of p-values from 0.05 to 0.0, our p-value is skewed to the right end.

0.05   0.001 0.0

A BF of 1.0 as computed in the current chapter looks very much incompatible with a p-value of 0.001. However, the underneath two lines give a more realistic pattern, because BFs run from ∞ to 0.0, and p-values run from 1.00 to 0.0. These lines show that they are very well compatible, and that they are indeed close to one another.

>100   1.0 0.0

1.00   0.05 0.0

With modern Bayesian statistics likelihood distribution rather than probability distribution modeling is used. It is mostly based on the Cauchy distribution, a member of the family of the alpha distributions, and the distribution that best describes the ratio of either two normal distributions or two likelihood distributions. Bayes factors have a Cauchy distribution, and can, therefore, not be numerically analyzed with standard Gaussian approximation methods. Fortunately, pretty good numerical results are obtained by integrations that integrate out nuisance variables. Nuisance variables are unwanted variables that increase overall variability in the data. Just like confounding variables, they tend not to differ between levels of independent variables. With binomial data, beta distributions are more adequate than normal distributions.

Suggested Reading[1,2]

Statistics applied to clinical studies 5th edition, 2012
Machine learning in medicine a complete overview, 2015
SPSS for starters and 2nd levelers 2nd edition, 2015
Clinical data analysis on a pocket calculator 2nd edition, 2016
Understanding clinical data analysis from published research, 2016
Modern meta-analysis, 2017
Regression Analysis in Clinical Research, 2018

---

[1] To readers requesting more background, theoretical and mathematical information of computations given, several textbooks complementary to the current production and written by the same authors are available.

[2] All of them have been written by the same authors, have been edited by Springer Heidelberg Germany.

Chapter 5
Bayesian Paired T-Test

5.1 Background

In studies with paired samples of continuous data the mean difference is usually compared to zero. They may be analyzed with the paired samples t-test, that is, if data can be assumed to follow a Gaussian-like pattern. The test assesses whether the mean difference and its 95% confidence interval (the alternative hypothesis H1) is significantly different from the value zero and the same 95% confidence interval (the null hypothesis H0). Instead of a paired t-test also a Bayesian analysis on the mean difference is possible. It assesses the magnitude of the Bayes factor (BF). A BF smaller than "one" supports the above alternative hypothesis (H1), while a BF larger than "one" supports the above null hypothesis (H0). The BF is computed as the ratio of two likelihood distributions, that of the posterior and the prior likelihood distribution. The first is modeled from the mode, the mean and standard deviation of the measured paired differences, the second is modeled from a conjugate pattern of the posterior (this is the same pattern as that of the posterior) but an uniformed uniform prior with a likelihood of "one" in the same interval as that of the posterior is pretty much OK as well. The computation of the BF requires integrations for accuracy purposes. But, then, it can be used as a statistical index to pretty precisely quantify the amount of support in favor H1 and H0. Advantages of the Bayesian approach may include.

1. A better underlying structure model of the H1 and H0 may be provided.
2. Maximal likelihoods of likelihood distributions are not always identical to the mean effect of traditional tests, and this may be fine, because biological likelihoods may better fit biological questions than numerical means of non-representative subgroups do.

However, in spite of this, nobody knows for sure why likelihood distributions may better than normal distributions estimate uncertainties in statistical test results. So, why not use both methods for analyzing the same data example. The current chapter will show and compare the results of traditional one sample t-tests and Bayesian one sample t-tests. For convenience a data file is in extras.springer.com and is entitled "chap5".

© Springer International Publishing AG, part of Springer Nature 2018
T. J. Cleophas, A. H. Zwinderman, *Modern Bayesian Statistics in Clinical Research*,
https://doi.org/10.1007/978-3-319-92747-3_5

5.2 Example

Start by opening the above data file in your computer loaded with SPSS statistical software version 25 including the module advanced statistics. In a 10 patient cross-over study the primary scientific question was: is the sleeping pill more efficacious than the placebo.

Var 1	2	3	4	5	6
6,1	5,2	54	0	0	0
7	7,9	55	0	0	0
8,2	3,9	78	1	0	0
7,6	4,7	53	1	1	1
6,5	5,3	49	1	1	1
8,4	5,4	85	1	1	1
6,9	4,2	77	0	1	1
6,7	6,1	66	0	1	1
7,4	3,8	79	0	0	1
5,8	6,3	67	1	0	1

Var 1 = hours of sleep during the use of a sleeping pill (Var = variable)
Var 2 = hours of sleep during placebo
Var 3 = age
Var 4 = gender
Var 5 = co-morbidity
Var 6 = co-medication

We will start with drawing a graph of the data.

Command:
click Graphs....click Bars....mark Summary Separate Variables....Define....Bars Represent....Options....SE 2....click OK.

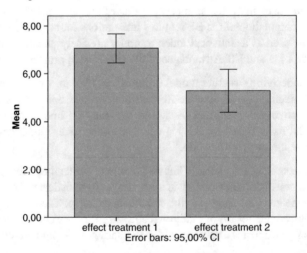

The above graph is in the output. The mean number of sleeping hours after sleeping pill seem to be larger than that after placebo. The whiskers represent the 95%

confidence intervals of the mean hours of sleep. They do not overlap, indicating that the difference between the two means is significant. The paired t-test can analyze the level of significance.

5.3   Traditional Analysis with Paired T-Test

Command:
Analyze....Compare Means....Paired Samples T-Test....Paired Variables: enter Variable 1: effect treatment 1....Variable 2: effect treatment 2....click OK.

Paired samples test

Paired differences

Mean	Std. deviation	Std. error mean	95% Confidence interval of the difference	
			Lower	Upper
1,78000	1,76811	,55913	,51517	3,04483

t	df	Sig. (2-tailed)
3,184	9	,011

The above tabling is in the output. The sleeping pill performs significantly better than does placebo with a p-value of 0.011, which is much smaller than 0.05. The difference is, thus, highly significant. The null hypothesis of no difference is rejected at a probability of 1.1%. We have 1.1% chance of a type I error of finding a difference where there is none. We can not conclude from this, that the alternative hypothesis is true, because this is a small study and type II and Type III errors may be involved. In order to better assess the real meaning of our data result and answering the question what chance we have, that the real effect is equally good, as it is from the traditional t-test, a Bayesian analysis will be performed. In addition to the Bayes factor and posterior likelihood distribution, in "Criteria" a 95% credible interval can be commanded. It may be wider than the traditional 95% confidence interval of the paired t-test, because a prior distribution are accounted. Also in "Priors" the type of prior setting can be commanded, either diffuse prior or Jeffreys prior.

5.4   Bayesian Analysis of Paired Continuous Data

Diffuse prior

Command:
Analyze....Bayesian Statistics....Related Samples Normal....Paired Variables: enter: Variable 1 effect treatment 1....variable 2 effect treatment 2....Bayesian Analysis: mark Use Both Methods....click Criteria: Credible interval percentage %: 95....click Continue....mark Priors: Validat....Diffuse....click Continue....click OK.

Bayes factor for one-sample T test

	N	Mean	Std. deviation	Std. error mean	Bayes factor	t	df	Sig. (2-tailed)
Effect treatment 1-effect treatment 2	10	1,7800	1,76811	,55913	0,178	3,184	9	0,011

Bayes factor, Null versus alternative hypothesis

Posterior distribution characterization for related-sample mean difference

	N	Posterior			95% Credible interval	
		Mode	Mean	Variance	Lower bound	Upper bound
Effect treatment 1-effect treatment 2	10	1,7800	1,7800	,563	,2809	3,2791

Prior on variance: diffuse. Prior on mean: diffuse

The above tables are in the output sheets. The upper table gives a Bayes factor of 0.178, which is <1.00 and so in support of a result in support of the alternative hypothesis, one treatment is better than the other. The lower table gives the 95% credible interval of the mean and mode of the posterior likelihood distribution.

Also in the output are the underneath three graphs.

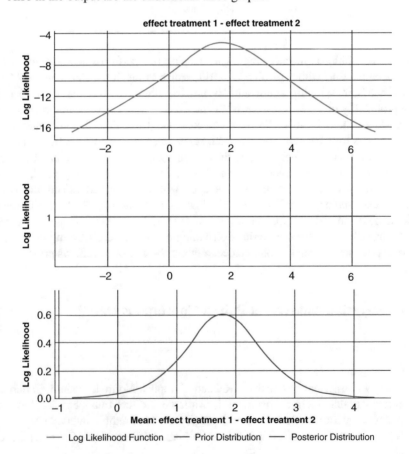

The above prior distribution is in red, it is uninformed and uniform with fx = 1 and an interval of approximately −2 to 6. The above posterior distribution is the likelihood distribution of the actual data results. It is in green with a mean of 1.78 h, and a maximum likelihood of 0.6. In blue the log transformation of the ratio of the blue and red curves is given with a maximal log (likelihood posterior/likelihood prior) = log (1.78/1) = 0.5108.

Bayes factor	Evidence category	Bayes factor	Evidence category	Bayes factor	Evidence category
>100	Extreme evidence for H0	1–3	Anecdotal evidence for H0	1/30 to 1/10	Strong evidence for H1
30–100	Very strong evidence for H0	1	No evidence	1/100 to 1/30	Very strong evidence for H1
10–30	Strong evidence for H0	1/3 to 1	Anecdotal evidence for H1	1/100	Extreme evidence for H1
3–10	Moderate evidence for H0	1/10 to 1/3	Moderate evidence for H1		

In the SPSS help-sheets available through the dialog boxes Bayes factor thresholds to define levels of support of H1 and H0. They have been reprinted above. The Bayes factor gives the ratio of the marginal likelihoods of the alternative hypothesis and the null hypothesis, and equals 0.178 in our example.

A BF of 0.178 would mean moderate support for the alternative hypothesis. The 95% credible interval, a Bayesian substitute for the confidence interval is a bit wider than the traditional 95% confidence interval of the means are, and the variance of the posterior mean is equally so as compared to the variance of the traditional t-test.

What does the Bayesian analysis tell, which we did not yet know. With traditional t tests we can only "yes or no" reject the null hypothesis. If not rejected, it does not mean the alternative hypothesis is true, because this is not assessed. It may very well be untrue, e.g., due to type II or III errors, or priors which changed the probability distribution of your outcome data. This is assessed with Bayesian analysis, and it can, therefore, tell us something about the alternative hypothesis, and also give us some more precise information, about how we should classify our estimates of the null hypothesis.

The Bayes factor (BF) in this chapter's example of 0.178 is compatible with the p-value of 0.011 as obtained from the traditional paired t-test.

On a continuous line of Bayes factors from 1.0 to 0.0, our Bayes factor is close to the right side end.

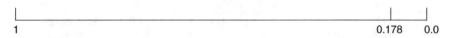

1   0.178   0.0

On a continuous line of p-values from 0.05 to 0.0 our p-value is similarly close to the right side end.

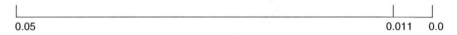

0.05   0.011   0.0

The BF of 0.178 is close to 0.0. Likewise a p-value of 0.011 is close to 0.0. The BF provides a statistic similar to that of the p-value.

Jeffreys prior

Prior distribution based on Jeffeys S2 or S4 give a bit better precisions than the above diffuse prior distribution do. Harold Jeffreys recommended that a "noninformant prior finding principle" should be invariant under monotone parameter transformation. The method is available in SPSS.

Commands:

Like the commands above, except in Priors: enter in Prior on Variance enter "Jeffreys 2", and in Prior on Mean enter "Diffuse".

Posterior distribution characterization for related-sample mean difference

	N	Posterior			95% Credible interval	
		Mode	Mean	Variance	Lower bound	Upper bound
Effect treatment 1-effect treatment 2	10	1,7800	1,7800	,402	,5152	3,0448

Prior on variance: Jeffreys 2. Prior on mean: diffuse

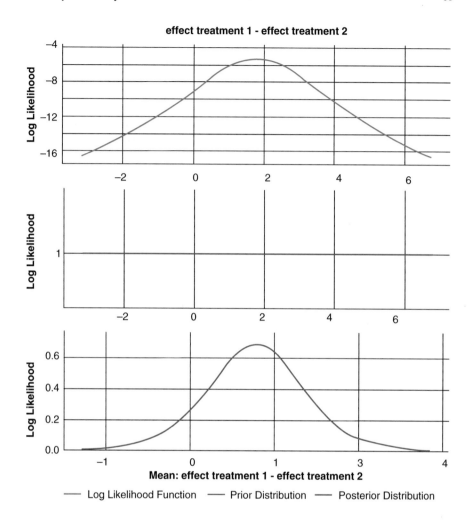

Commands:
Like the commands above, except in Priors: enter in Prior on Variance enter "Jeffreys 4", and in Prior on Mean enter "Diffuse".

Posterior distribution characterization for related-sample mean difference

	N	Posterior			95% Credible interval	
		Mode	Mean	Variance	Lower bound	Upper bound
Effect treatment 1-effect treatment 2	10	1,7800	1,7800	,313	,6669	2,8931

Prior on variance: Jeffreys 4. Prior on mean: diffuse

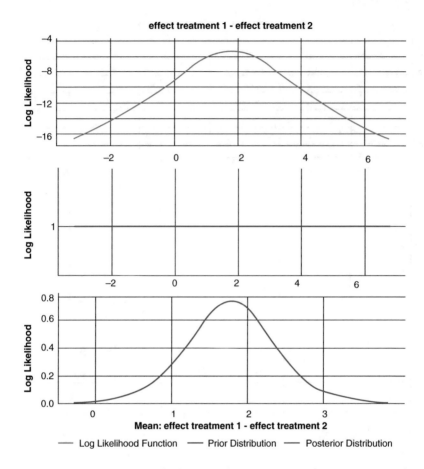

— Log Likelihood Function — Prior Distribution — Posterior Distribution

The above tables and graphs comparing a diffuse prior with two types of Jeffreys priors show that the credible intervals of the get better and better. The Jeffreys 2 and particularly 4 have narrower intervals, and, so, give better precisions than the diffuse prior does:

	95% credible interval
1 uniform prior	0.2809–3.2791
2 Jeffreys 2 prior	0.5152–3.0498
3 Jeffreys 4 prior	0.6699–2.8931.

5.5 Conclusion

This chapter assesses the Bayesian paired t-test. The results are pretty similar to those of the traditional paired t-test. The Bayesian t-test provides less precision in support of the alternative hypothesis than the traditional t-test does. However, with Jeffreys priors precision is considerably improved.

Advantages of the Bayesian approach may include.

1. A better underlying structure of the H1 and H0 may be provided.
2. Bayesian tests work with 95% credible intervals that are usually somewhat wider and this may reduce the chance of statistical significances with little clinical relevance.
3. Maximal likelihoods of likelihood distributions are not always identical to the mean effect of traditional tests, and this may be fine, because biological likelihoods may better fit biological questions than numerical means of non-representative subgroups do.
4. Bayes uses ratios of likelihood distributions rather than ratios of Gaussian distributions, which are notorious for ill data fit.
5. Bayesian integral computations are very advanced, and, therefore, give optimal precisions of complex functions, and better so than traditional multiple mean calculations of non representative subsamples do.
6. with Bayesian testing type I and II errors need not being taken into account.

A disadvantage of Bayesian methods may be overfitting. This means that the likelihood distributions are wider than compatible Gaussian modeling. Bootstraps t-test is based on Monte Carlo resampling from your own data. It is available in SPSS statistical software. In the example given we will compare a bootstraps sampling distribution in SPSS with Bayesian likelihood and traditional Gaussian distributions.

Open once more the data file entitled "chap5" stored at extras.springer.com in your personal computer mounted with SPSS.

Command:
Analyze....Compare Means....Paired Samples T Test....Dialog Box....Paired Variables....Variable 1 enter effect treatment 1....Variable 2 enter effect treatment 2....click Bootstrap....click Perform bootstrapping....Number Samples enter 1000....click Continue....click OK.

The bootstrap resampling model is in the output sheets and it provides a 95% confidence interval between 0.76025 and 2.8400.

The Bayesian and traditional t-test 95% confidence intervals are given above.

1. Traditional t-test 95% confidence interval between 0.51517 and 3.04483
2. Bootstraps t-test 95% confidence interval between 0.76025 and 2.8400
3. Bayesian t-test 95% credible interval between 0.2809 and 3.2791.

The traditional t-test confidence interval is wider than the bootstraps t-test confidence interval, while the Bayesian 95% credible interval is the widest.

Some overfitting in the traditional and Bayesian intervals can not be excluded, and in the Bayesian this may be more so than in the traditional. Nonetheless the amount of overfitting is limited with confidence intervals between ≈ 2.3 and ≈ 2.8.

Suggested Reading[1,2]

Statistics applied to clinical studies 5th edition, 2012
Machine learning in medicine a complete overview, 2015
SPSS for starters and 2nd levelers 2nd edition, 2015
Clinical data analysis on a pocket calculator 2nd edition, 2016
Understanding clinical data analysis from published research, 2016
Modern Meta-analysis, 2017
Regression Analysis in Clinical Research, 2018

---

[1] To readers requesting more background, theoretical and mathematical information of computations given, several textbooks complementary to the current production and written by the same authors are available.

[2] All of them have been written by the same authors, and have been edited by Springer Heidelberg Germany.

Chapter 6
Bayesian Unpaired T-Test

6.1 Background

In studies with two unpaired samples of continuous data the difference of the two means and their pooled standard error is usually compared to zero. These studies may be analyzed with the unpaired samples t-test, that is, if data can be assumed to follow a Gaussian-like pattern. The test assesses whether the difference of the two means and its pooled 95% confidence interval (the alternative hypothesis, H1) is significantly different from the value zero and the same pooled 95% confidence interval (the null hypothesis, H0). Instead of an unpaired t-test also a Bayesian analysis on the difference of two group means is possible. It assesses the likelihood distribution of the measured data (the posterior likelihood distribution) adjusted for an informed prior likelihood distribution. If the latter is not available, either (1) two identical uninformed priors for both treatment groups, or (2) two reference priors adjusted for difference in variances of the two groups (reference means here equal to standard gamma distributions) can be applied instead. The unpaired Bayesian analysis assesses the magnitude of the ratio of the posterior and the prior, and is otherwise called the Bayes factor (BF). A BF smaller than "one" supports the above alternative hypothesis (H1), while a BF larger than "one" supports the above null hypothesis (H0). The posterior is modeled from the mean and standard deviation of the measured unpaired differences, the second can be modeled either from the above uniformed priors or from the above reference priors. The computation of the BF requires integrations for accuracy purposes. But, then, it can be used as a statistical index to pretty precisely quantify the amount of support in favor H1 (the difference between the unpaired means is larger than zero), and H0 (the difference between the unpaired means is not larger than zero). Advantages of the Bayesian approach may include.

1. A better underlying structure model of the H1 and H0 may be provided.
2. Maximal likelihoods of likelihood distributions are not always identical to the mean effect of traditional tests, and this may be fine, because biological

© Springer International Publishing AG, part of Springer Nature 2018
T. J. Cleophas, A. H. Zwinderman, *Modern Bayesian Statistics in Clinical Research*,
https://doi.org/10.1007/978-3-319-92747-3_6

likelihoods may better fit biological questions than numerical means of non-representative subgroups do.

However, in spite of this, nobody knows for sure why likelihood distributions may better than normal distributions estimate uncertainties in statistical test results. So, why not use both methods for analyzing the same data example. The current chapter will show and compare the results of traditional unpaired t-tests and Bayesian alternatives, currently called Bayesian unpaired t-tests. For convenience a data file is in extras.springer.com, and is entitled "chap6".

6.2 Example

Start by opening the data file in your computer loaded with SPSS statistical software version 25 the module advanced statistics included. The primary scientific question of a 20 patient parallel group study of effect assesses whether a sleeping pill is more efficacious than a placebo with hours of sleep as outcome variable.

Var				
1	2	3	4	5
0	6	45	0	1
0	7,1	45	0	1
0	8,1	46	0	0
0	7,5	37	0	0
0	6,4	48	0	1
0	7,9	76	1	1
0	6,8	56	1	1
0	6,6	54	1	0
0	7,3	63	1	0
0	5,6	75	0	0
1	5,1	64	1	0
1	8	35	0	1
1	3,8	46	1	0
1	4,4	44	0	1
1	5,2	64	1	0
1	5,4	75	0	1
1	4,3	65	1	1
1	6	84	1	0
1	3,7	35	1	0
1	6,2	46	0	1

Var = variable
Var 1 = group 0 has placebo, group 1 has sleeping pill
Var 2 = hours of sleep
Var 3 = age
Var 4 = gender
Var 5 = co-morbidity

6.3   Traditional Unpaired T-Test

Open the data file stored at extras.springer.com and entitled "chap6" in your computer mounted SPSS version 25 with the module advanced statistics included.

Command:
Analyze....Compare Means....Independent Samples T Test....Dialog Box....
Grouping Variable: enter Group 1 : 1....Group 2: 0....click Continue....click OK.

Group statistics

	Group	N	Mean	Std. deviation	Std. error mean
Effect treatment	1.00	10	5.2100	1.29910	0.41081
	0.00	10	6.9300	0.80561	0.25475

Independent samples test

		Levene's test for equality of variances		t-test for equality of means					95% Confidence interval of the difference	
		F	Sig.	t	df	Sig. (2-tailed)	Mean difference	Std. error difference	Lower	Upper
Effect treatment	Equal variances assumed	1.060	0.317	−3.558	18	0.002	−1.72000	0.48339	−2.73557	−0.70443
	Equal variances not assumed			−3.558	15.030	0.003	−1.72000	0.48339	−2.75014	−0.68986

The above tables are in the output sheets. The unpaired t-test shows that a significant difference exists between the sleeping pill and the placebo with a p-value of 0.002 or 0.003. Generally, it is better to use the largest of the p-values given, because the smallest p-value makes assumptions that are not always warranted, like, for example, in the above table, the presence of equal variances of the means of variables 1 and 2. The sleeping pill performs significantly better than does placebo, with p-values much smaller than 0.05. The difference is, thus, highly significant. The null hypothesis of no difference is rejected at a probability 0.002 or 0.003. We have 0.2 or 0.3% chance of a type I error of finding a difference where there is none. We can not conclude from this, that the alternative hypothesis is true, because this is a small study and type I and Type II errors may be involved. Moreover, strictly, null hypothesis testing does not allow making conclusions about the alternative hypothesis H1. In order to try and find support for both the null and the alternative hypotheses, a Bayesian t-test will be performed. The submodule Bayesian Statistics in Advanced Statistics must be used. In addition to Bayes factors and posterior likelihood distributions, in "Criteria" given in the dialog boxes 95% credible intervals will be measured. They may tend to be wider than the traditional 95% confidence intervals, because prior distributions are accounted. In "Priors" the type of prior setting can be commanded. Here we will mark, that Rouder's method will be used. Rouder's method uses subsets of data from a variable rather than the overall data for estimating frequency distributions.

6.4 Bayesian Unpaired T-Test

Command:
Analyze....Bayesian Statistics....Independent Samples Normal....Test Variable(s): enter effect treatment....Grouping Variable: enter "group"....Define Groups: Group 1: 0....Group 2: 1.... Bayesian Analysis: mark Use Both Methods....click Criteria: Credible interval percentage %: 95....click Continue....click Priors: click Assume unequal variances....click OK.

Group statistics

	Group	N	Mean	Std. deviation	Std. error mean
Effect treatmet	=0.00	10	6.9300	0.80561	0.25475
	=1.00	10	5.2100	1.29910	0.41081

Bayes factor independent sample test (Method = Rouder)[a]

	Mean difference	Pooled std. error difference	Bayes factor[b]	t	df	Sig. (2-tailed)
Effect treatment	−1.7200	0.48339	0.056	−3.558	18	0.002

[a]Assumes unequal variance between groups
[b]Bayes factor: null versus alternative hypothesis

Posterior distribution characterization for independent sample mean[a]

	Posterior			95% Credible interval	
	Mode	Mean	Variance	Lower bound	Upper bound
Effect treatment	−1.7200	−1.7200	0.300	−2.8098	−0.6302

[a]Prior for variance: diffuse. Prior for mean: diffuse

The above tables in the output sheets show that a Bayes factor <1.0 is computed, suggesting that the traditional alternative hypothesis is supported. Also the 95% credible interval of the posterior likelihood distribution between −2.8098 and −0.6302 is given.

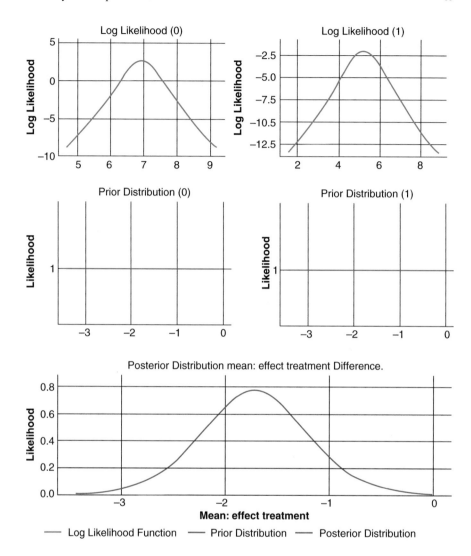

The above three graphs are also given in the output sheets.

The prior distributions in red are two, one for either of the unpaired groups (group 0 and group 1). They are noninformative and uniform, with f x = 1, and an interval between approximately −3 and 0. It may seem unbelievable but it works. The above posterior distribution, the likelihood distribution of the actual data results is in green with a mean of −1.72 h, and a maximum likelihood of 0.8. In blue, instead of a single, two log likelihood distributions are given one of the zero treatment data and one of the one treatment data. As shown diffuse priors were used for unknown variances assumed to be unequal. For computations marginal posterior distributions are integrated out.

The credible interval of the Bayesian test is wider than the 95% confidence of the traditional t-test is, −2.8098 to −0.6302 as compared to −2.75014 to −0.68986. And so less precision is given with Bayes.

The Bayes factor (BF) in this chapter's example of 0.056 is compatible with the p-value of 0.002 as obtained from the traditional paired t-test.

On a continuous line of Bayes factors from 1.0 to 0.0, our Bayes factor is close to the right side end.

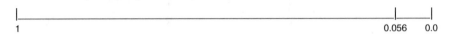

On a continuous line of p-values from 0.05 to 0.0 our p-value is similarly close to the right side end.

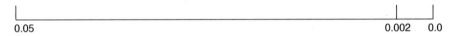

The underneath Bayes factor table, available in the SPSS help-sheets, similarly shows that a Bayes factor of 0.056 supports for the alternative hypothesis, a true difference between placebo and sleeping pill. This result thus supports the traditional t-test.

Bayes factor	Evidence category	Bayes factor	Evidence category	B-ayes factor	Evidence category
>100	Extreme evidence for H0	1–3	Anecdotal evidence for H0	1/30 to 1/10	Strong evidence for H1
30–100	Very strong evidence for H0	1	No evidence	1/100 to 1/30	Very strong evidence for H1
10–30	Strong evidence for H0	1/3 to 1	Anecdotal evidence for H1	1/100	Extreme evidence for H1
3–10	Moderate evidence for H0	1/10 to 1/3	Moderate evidence for H1		

6.5   Bayesian Unpaired T-Test with Informed Prior: Variance per Group Adjusted

A Bayesian Unpaired T-test with Informed Prior will be performed. For the purpose the data were adjusted for variances per group. The above commands will be given once more, but now with variances of separate groups added as additional information a priori demonstrated in a similar historical trial (group 0 variance 0.64, group 1 variance 1.69).

Command:

Analyze....Bayesian Statistics....Independent Samples Normal....Test Variable(s): enter effect treatment....Grouping Variable: enter "group"....Define Groups: Group 1: 0....Group 2: 1.... Bayesian Analysis: mark Use Both Methods....click Criteria: Credible interval percentage %: 95....click Continue....click Priors: Variance known: Group 1 variance: enter 0,64....Group 2 variance: enter 1,69.... click Continue....click OK.

Group statistics

	Group	N	Mean	Std. deviation	Std. error mean
Effect treatmet	=0.00	10	6.9300	0.80561	0.25475
	=1.00	10	5.2100	1.29910	0.41081

Bayes factor independent sample 3 (Method = Rouder)[a]

	Mean difference	Pooled std. error difference	Bayes factor[b]	t	df	Sig. (2-tailed)
Effect treatment	−1.7200	0.48339	0.056	−3.558	18	0.002

[a]Assumes unequal variance between groups
[b]Bayes factor: null versus alternative hypothesis

Posterior distribution characterization for independent sample mean[a]

	Posterior			95% Credible interval	
	Mode	Mean	Variance	Lower bound	Upper bound
Effect treatment	−1.7200	−1.7200	0.300	−2.8098	−0.6302

[a]Prior for variance: diffuse. Prior for mean: normal

The above three tables are in the output. Like with the uninformed model the BF is 0.056. However, the posterior mean and mode are different, −1.9719 instead of −1.7200. Also the credible intervals are so, −2.8587 to −1.0851, instead of −2.8098 to −0.6302.

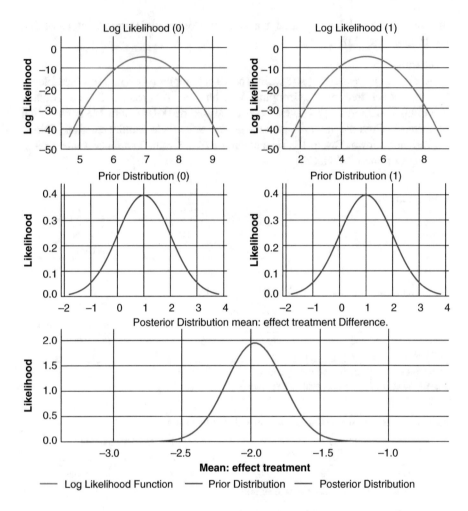

The above three graphs also in the output. As compared to the previous graphs we now have two informed prior likelihood distributions instead of two diffuse priors.

If we have prior information available, like in this case the variance in the two groups, this information can be entered in the prior information dialog box. The noninformative prior distribution is then changed into curves based on this prior information. It has a substantial effect on the outcome. We should add that the sample is small, with large samples the effect of prior information rapidly wears off. At the same time, the 95% credible interval of the posterior likelihood distribution decreases: -2.858 to -1.0851 instead of -2.8098 to -0.6302. Better precision is, thus, provided with an interval of 1.7729 instead of 2.1796.

6.6   Conclusion

This chapter assesses the Bayesian unpaired t-test. The results are pretty similar to those of the traditional unpaired t-test. The Bayesian unpaired test provides slightly less precision in support of the alternative hypothesis if uniformed and slightly better if informed, as compared to the traditional unpaired t-test.

The above Bayes factor table given by SPSS is drawn underneath with a red diagonal line added. It may be helpful to distinguish positive and negative studies.

Reject H1

Bayes Factor	Evidence Category	Bayes Factor	Evidence Category	Bayes Factor	Evidence Category
>100	Extreme Evidence for H0	1-3	Anecdotal Evidence for H0	1/30-1/10	Strong Evidence for H1
30-100	Very Strong Evidence for H0	1	No Evidence	1/100-1/30	VeryStrong Evidence for H1
10-30	Strong Evidence for H0	1/3-1	Anecdotal Evidence for H1	1/100	Extreme Evidence for H1
3-10	Moderate Evidence for H0	1/10-1/3	Moderate Evidence for H1		

Reject H0

Advantages of the Bayesian approach may include.

1. A better underlying structure of the H1 and H0 may be provided.
2. Bayesian tests work with 95% credible intervals that are usually somewhat wider and this may reduce the chance of statistical significances with little clinical relevance.
3. Maximal likelihoods of likelihood distributions are not always identical to the mean effect of traditional tests, and this may be fine, because biological likelihoods may better fit biological questions than numerical means of non-representative subgroups do.
4. Bayes uses ratios of likelihood distributions rather than ratios of Gaussian distributions, which are notorious for ill data fit.
5. Bayesian integral computations are very advanced, and, therefore, give optimal precisions of complex functions, and better so than traditional multiple mean calculations of non representative subsamples do.
6. With Bayesian testing type I and II errors need not being taken into account.

A disadvantage of Bayesian methods may be overfitting. This means that the likelihood distributions are wider than compatible Gaussian modeling. Bootstraps t-test is based on Monte Carlo resampling from your own data. It is available in SPSS statistical software. In the example given we will compare a bootstraps sampling distribution in SPSS with Bayesian likelihood and traditional Gaussian distributions.

Open the data file entitled "chap6" stored at extras.springer.com in your personal computer mounted with SPSS.

Command:
Analyze....Compare Means....Independent Samples T Test....Dialog Box.... Grouping Variable: enter Group 1 : 1....Group 2: 0....click Bootstrap....click Perform bootstrapping....Number Samples enter 1000....click Continue....click OK.

The underneath tables are in the output sheets. The bootstrap resampling model provides a 95% confidence interval between −2.61536 and −0.71752.

The Bayesian and traditional t-test 95% confidence intervals are given underneath.

1. Bootstraps unpaired t-test 95% confidence interval	−2.61536 to −0.71752
2. Bayesian unpaired t-test 95% credible interval	−2.80980 to −0.63020
3. Gaussian unpaired t-test 95% confidence interval	−2.73557 to −0.79443

Obviously the 95% confidence interval of the bootstraps t-test is closer to the traditional Gaussian t-test than it is to the Bayesian t-test. Under the assumption that bootstrap sampling is entirely without overfitting, this would be an argument of overfitting of the Bayesian t-test and an argument in favor of the traditional Gaussian approach. However, with the above informed prior example this was less a problem.

Suggested Reading[1,2]

Statistics applied to clinical studies 5th edition, 2012
Machine learning in medicine a complete overview, 2015
SPSS for starters and 2nd levelers 2nd edition, 2015
Clinical data analysis on a pocket calculator 2nd edition, 2016
Understanding clinical data analysis from published research, 2016
Modern Meta-analysis, 2017
Regression Analysis in Clinical Research, 2018

---

[1] To readers requesting more background, theoretical and mathematical information of computations given, several textbooks complementary to the current production and written by the same authors are available.

[2] All of them have been written by the same authors and they have been edited by Springer Heidelberg Germany.

Chapter 7
Bayesian Regressions

7.1 Background

In studies with two unpaired samples of continuous data as outcome and a binary predictor like treatment modality the difference of the two means and their pooled standard error is usually compared to zero. These studies may be analyzed with linear regression, that is, if data can be assumed to follow Gaussian-like patterns. The analysis assesses whether (1) the correlation coefficient is significantly larger than zero (using analysis of variance) or (2) the difference of the two means and its pooled 95% confidence interval (the alternative hypothesis, H1) is significantly different from the value zero and the same pooled 95% confidence interval (the null hypothesis, H0) (using the t-test). Instead of the above tests a Bayesian regression analysis is possible.

It assesses the magnitude of the Bayes factors computed from the ratio of the posterior and prior likelihood distribution. The posterior is modeled from the mean and variance of the measured unpaired differences, the prior is usually modeled as an uninformative prior either from the Jeffreys Zellner Siow (JZS) method or, equivalently, from the computation of a reference prior based on a gamma distribution with a standard error of "1". The computation of the BF requires integrations for accuracy purposes. But, then, it can be used as a statistical index to pretty precisely quantify the amount of support in favor H1 (the difference between the unpaired means is larger than zero), and H0 (the difference between the unpaired means is not larger than zero). Advantages of the Bayesian approach may include.

1. A better underlying structure model of the H1 and H0 may be provided.
2. Maximal likelihoods of likelihood distributions are not always identical to the mean effect of traditional tests, and this may be fine, because biological likelihoods may better fit biological questions than numerical means of non-representative subgroups do.

© Springer International Publishing AG, part of Springer Nature 2018   69
T. J. Cleophas, A. H. Zwinderman, *Modern Bayesian Statistics in Clinical Research*,
https://doi.org/10.1007/978-3-319-92747-3_7

However, in spite of this, nobody knows for sure why likelihood distributions may better than normal distributions estimate uncertainties in statistical test results. So, why not use both methods for analyzing the same data example. The current chapter will show and compare the results of traditional linear regression with that of Bayesian linear regression. For convenience a data file is in extras.springer.com, and is entitled "chap7".

7.2   Introduction, Data Example

Start by opening the data file in your computer with SPSS statistical software version 25 mounted including the module advanced statistics. The data are given underneath.

Variable				
1	2	3	4	5
0,00	6,00	65,00	0,00	1,00
0,00	7,10	75,00	0,00	1,00
0,00	8,10	86,00	0,00	0,00
0,00	7,50	74,00	0,00	0,00
0,00	6,40	64,00	0,00	1,00
0,00	7,90	75,00	1,00	1,00
0,00	6,80	65,00	1,00	1,00
0,00	6,60	64,00	1,00	0,00
0,00	7,30	75,00	1,00	0,00
0,00	5,60	56,00	0,00	0,00
1,00	5,10	55,00	1,00	0,00
1,00	8,00	85,00	0,00	1,00
1,00	3,80	36,00	1,00	0,00
1,00	4,40	47,00	0,00	1,00
1,00	5,20	58,00	1,00	0,00
1,00	5,40	56,00	0,00	1,00
1,00	4,30	46,00	1,00	1,00
1,00	6,00	64,00	1,00	0,00
1,00	3,70	33,00	1,00	0,00
1,00	6,20	65,00	0,00	1,00

Var 1 = group 0 has placebo, group 1 has sleeping pill
Var 2 = hours of sleep
Var 3 = age
Var 4 = gender
Var 5 = co-morbidity

The above table are the data of a 20 patient parallel group study of two groups assessed for hours of sleep after treatment with a placebo (0) or a sleeping pill (1). Similarly to an unpaired t-test, linear regression can be used to test whether there is a significant difference between two treatment modalities. To see how it works picture a linear regression of hours of sleep and treatment modalities. It may show that the better the treatment modality, the more hours of sleep will be observed. Treatment modalities are drawn on the x-axis, hours of sleep on the y-axis, and the best fit regression line about the data can be calculated, and is given underneath.

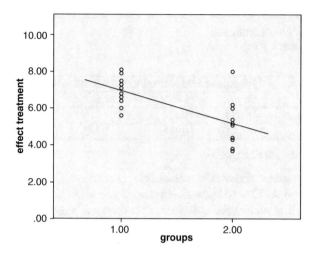

As shown, instead of a continuous variable on the x-axis, a binary variable can be adequately used, e.g., two treatment modalities, a bad and a good treatment. With hours of sleep on the y-axis, a nice linear regression analysis can be performed: the better the sleeping treatment, the larger the numbers of sleeping hours. The treatment modality is called the x-variable, or independent variable, or exposure variable, or predictor variable, the hours of sleep is called the y-variable, or dependent variable or outcome variable. For convenience, the data are given in extras.springer.com, and are entitled "chap7". With SPSS statistical software the underneath parameters are obtained from a linear regression of these data using just two variables, hours of sleep as outcome and treatment modality as predictor. The commands are given underneath.

7.3   Traditional Linear Regression Analysis

Command:
Analyze....Regression....Linear....Dependent: treatment effect....Independent: group....click OK.

The underneath tables are in the output sheets.
Model summary

Model	R	R square	Adjusted R square	Std. error of the estimate
1	0.643[a]	0.413	0.380	1.08089

[a]Predictors: (constant), group

ANOVA[a]

Model		Sum of squares	df	Mean square	F	Sig.
1	Regression	14,792	1	14,792	12.661	0.002[b]
	Residual	21,030	18	1,168		
	Total	35,822	19			

[a]Dependent variable: effect treatment
[b]Predictors: (constant), group

Coefficients[a]

Model		Unstandardized coefficients		Standardized coefficients		
		B	Std. error	Beta	t	Sig.
1	(Constant)	6.930	0.342		20.274	0.000
	Group	−1.720	0.483	−0.643	−3.558	0.002

[a]Dependent variable: effect treatment

The upper table shows the correlation coefficient (R = 0.643 = 64%). R-square = R^2 = 0.413 = 41%, meaning that, if you know the treatment modality, you will be able to predict the treatment effect (hours of sleep) with 41% certainty. You will then be uncertain with 59% uncertainty. The magnitude of the R-value is important for making predictions. However, the size of the study sample is also important: with a sample of say three subjects little prediction is possible. This is, particularly, assessed in the middle table. It tests with analysis of variance (ANOVA) whether there is a significant correlation between the x and y-variables.

It does so by assessing whether the calculated R-square value is significantly different from an R-square value of 0. The answer is yes. The p-value equals 0.002, and, so, the treatment modality is a significant predictor of the treatment modality.

The bottom table shows the calculated B-value (the regression coefficient). The B-value is obtained by counting/multiplying the individual data values, and it behaves in the regression model as a kind of mean result. Like many mean values from random data samples, this also means, that the B-value can be assumed to follow a Gaussian distribution, and that it can, therefore, be assessed with a t-test. The calculated t-value from these data is smaller than −1.96, namely −3.558, and, therefore, the p-value is <0.05. The interpretation of this finding is, approximately, the same as the interpretation of the R-square value: a significant B-value means that B is significantly larger or smaller (like here) than 0, and, thus, that the x-variable is a significant predictor of the y-variable. If you square the t-value, and compare it with the F-value of the ANOVA table, then you will observe that the values are identical. The two tests are, indeed, largely similar. One of the two tests is somewhat redundant.

Not only treatment modality, but also patient characteristics like age, gender, and co-morbidity may be significant predictors of hours of sleep. An interesting thing about regression analysis is that, in addition to treatment modality, such characteristics can be included in the model as predictor variables.

In the example given, the null hypothesis of a B value not significantly different from zero is rejected at a probability of 0.002 = 0.2%. We have 0.2%

chance of a type I error of finding a difference where there is none. We can not conclude from this, that the alternative hypothesis, that our result is not significantly different from the measured B ± its SE, is true, because this was not assessed. In order to answer the question what level of likelihood we have to support either the null (H0) or the alternative hypothesis (H1), a modern Bayesian linear regression analysis will be performed. For that purpose, in SPSS statistical software module version 25 (2017) loaded with the module advanced statistics, a Bayesian linear regression analysis will be performed. Start by opening the data file entitled "chap7" once more in your computer stored with the above SPSS statistical software.

7.4   Bayesian Linear Regression Analysis

Command:
click in Menu: Analyze....Bayesian Statistics....Linear Regression....Dependent: effect treatment....Covariate(s): group....Bayesian Analysis: mark Use Both Methods....click Criteria: Credible interval percentage %: 95....click Continue.... click Priors: mark Reference priors, otherwise like the default version....click Continue....click OK.

Note, unlike with unpaired and paired t-tests one sample tests the Bayes factor is not computed with "supporting null versus alternative hypothesis" but, in contrast, with the other way around. Why so? Regressions are usually explorative, and multiple Bayes factors are used for comparing the results. Large Bayes factors (BFs) may be more convenient for comparisons than small ones, but, otherwise, this is not a necessity. In so doing very large BFs will support the traditional alternative, and very small BFs will support the traditional null hypothesis.

The underneath tables are in the output sheets.

ANOVA[a,b]

Source	Sum of squares	df	Mean square	F	Sig.
Regression	14,792	1	14,792	12.661	0.002
Residual	21,030	18	1,168		
Total	35,822	19			

[a]Dependent variable: effect treatment
[b]Model: (intercept), group

Bayes factor model summary[a,b]

Bayes factor	R	R square	Adjusted R square	Std. error of the estimate
17.329	0.643	0.413	0.380	1.0809

[a]Method: JZS
[b]Model: (intercept), group

Bayesian estimates of coefficients[a,b,c]

Parameter	Posterior			95% Credible interval	
	Mode	Mean	Variance	Lower bound	Upper bound
(Intercept)	5.210	5.210	0.131	4.492	5.928
Group = 0.00	1,720	1,720	,263	,704	2.736
Group = 1.00	d	d	d	d	d

[a]Dependent variable: effect treatment
[b]Model: (intercept), group
[c]Assume standard reference priors
[d]This parameter is redundant. Posterior statistics are not calculated

Bayesian estimates of error variance[a]

Parameter	Posterior			95% Credible interval	
	Mode	Mean	Variance	Lower bound	Upper bound
Error variance	1.052	1.314	0.247	0.667	2.555

[a]Assume standard reference priors

The first table above is identical to the ANOVA table of the traditional regressions analysis. The second table gives the Bayes factor. It is computed from the likelihood sum of posterior and prior likelihood distributions where posterior and prior are based on alternative and null hypothesis. For computing the prior likelihood distribution the null hypothesis is used with the help of the JZS (Jeffrey Zellner Siow) method. It is a way for computing priors equivalent to those computed with standard beta (for binomial data) and gamma (for continuous and normal data) distributions with a standard error of 1. It is usually named reference priors because of its reference to the standard data distributions. These priors are adequate for Bayesian linear regressions and Bayesian analyses of variance with. otherwise, lacking informative priors. The footnote "c" confirms that support of H1 is assessed versus that of null, and, not like in the previous four chapters, the other way around. And so, the computed very large BF of over >17.0 suggests that H1 is supported and H0 is not so. The underneath table as modified from SPSS's help pages gives patterns and meanings.

Reject H0

Bayes Factor	Evidence Category	Bayes Factor	Evidence Category	Bayes Factor	Evidence Category
>100	Extreme Evidence for H1	1-3	Anecdotal Evidence for H1	1/30-1/10	Strong Evidence for H0
30-100	Very Strong Evidence for H1	1	No Evidence	1/100-1/30	Very Strong Evidence for H0
10-30	Strong Evidence for H1	1/3-1	Anecdotal Evidence for H0	1/100	Extreme Evidence for H0
3-10	Moderate Evidence for H1	1/10-1/3	Moderate Evidence for H0		

Reject H1

With regression analysis and analysis of variance, which is actually just another kind of regression analysis with dependent and independent variables, multiple predictor variables are often added to the analysis in order to explore and find the best fit combination of variables. With many predictors, however, statistical power is lost. With Bayesian statistics this is observed as increasingly smaller BFs. The above Bayesian Estimates of Coefficients table gives Bayesian coefficients in the form of means, modes and credible intervals. The values are obviously slightly different from those of the traditional regression coefficients, particularly the traditional 95% confidence values are different from the 95% credible interval, a Bayesian substitute for the 95% confidence interval. It is a bit wider, between 0.704 and 2.736 as compared to 0.754 and 2.685 for the traditional linear regression.

The Bayes factor (BF) in this example of 17.329 is compatible with the p-value of 0.02 as obtained from the traditional linear regression.

On a continuous line of Bayes factors from >30 to 1.0, our Bayes factor is not far from the middle.

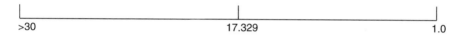

On a continuous line of p-values from 0.0 to 0.05 our p-value is similarly not far from the middle.

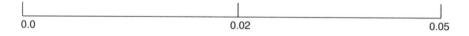

Reject H0

Bayes Factor	Evidence Category	Bayes Factor	Evidence Category	Bayes Factor	Evidence Category
>100	Extreme Evidence for H1	1-3	Anecdotal Evidence for H1	1/30-1/10	Strong Evidence for H0
30-100	Very Strong Evidence for H1	1	No Evidence	1/100-1/30	Very Strong Evidence for H0
10-30	Strong Evidence for H1	1/3-1	Anecdotal Evidence for H0	1/100	Extreme Evidence for H0
3-10	Moderate Evidence for H1	1/10-1/3	Moderate Evidence for H0		

Reject H1

The above Bayes factor table underscores that a Bayes factor of 17.329 strongly supports the alternative hypothesis, a true difference between placebo and sleeping pill. This result, thus, supports that of the traditional t-test. And so, a Bayes factor of 17.329 gives strong support not only in favor of the alternative hypothesis but also against the null hypothesis.

7.5 Traditional Multiple Linear Regression Analysis with Binary Predictors

With traditional regression analysis and three binary predictors instead of a single one, the non significant predictors are traditionally considered to be meaningless, and removed from the model. The above example will used once more but now with three instead of a single predictor variable. The same data example is used once more.

Command:
Analyze....Regression....Linear....Dependent: treatment effect....Independent: group, male/female, comorbidity....click OK.

Model summary

Model	R	R square	Adjusted R square	Std. error of the estimate
1	0.669[a]	0.448	0.345	1.11169

[a]Predictors: (constant), comorbidity, group, male/female

ANOW[a]

Model		Sum of squares	df	Mean square	F	Sig.
1	Regression	16,048	3	5,349	4.329	0.021[b]
	Residual	19,774	16	1,236		
	Total	35,822	19			

[a]Dependent variable: effect treatment
[b]Predictors: (constant), comorbidity, group, male/female

Coefficients[a]

Model		Unstandardized coefficients		Standardized coefficients		
		B	Std. error	Beta	t	Sig.
1	(Constant)	6.984	0.545		12.824	0.000
	Group	−1.642	0.509	−0.613	−3.223	0.005
	Male/female	−0.390	0.556	−0.146	−0.702	0.493
	Comorbidity	0.204	0.545	0.076	0.375	0.713

[a]Dependent variable: effect treatment

The above tables show that the added variables gender and comorbidity are not significantly different from zero, and may, therefore, be defined as meaningless, and be removed from the analysis.

7.6 Bayesian Multiple Linear Regression Analysis

Command:
click in Menu: Analyze....Bayesian Statistics....Linear Regression....Dependent: effect treatment....Covariate(s): group, male/female, comorbidity....Bayesian Analysis: mark Use Both Methods....click Criteria: Credible interval percentage %: 95....click Continue....click Priors: mark Reference priors....click Continue.... click OK.

The underneath four tables are in the output sheets.

ANOVA[a,b]

Source	Sum of squares	df	Mean square	F	Sig.
Regression	16,048	3	5,349	4.329	0.021
Residual	19,774	16	1,236		
Total	35,822	19			

[a]Dependent variable: effect treatment
[b]Model: (intercept), group, male/female, comorbidity

Bayes factor model summary[a,b]

Bayes factor[c]	R	R square	Adjusted R square	Std. error of the estimate
1.626	0.669	0.448	0.345	1.1117

[a]Method: JZS
[b]Model: (intercept), group, male/female, comorbidity
[c]Bayes factor: testing model versus null model (intercept)

Bayesian estimates of coefficients[a,b,c]

Parameter	Posterior			95% Credible interval	
	Mode	Mean	Variance	Lower bound	Upper bound
(Intercept)	5.156	5.156	0.339	4.001	6.311
Group = 1.00	1.642	1.642	0.297	0.562	2.722
Group = 1.00	d	d	d	d	d
Male/female = 0.00	0.390	0.390	0.353	−0.788	1.568
Male/female = 1.00	d.	d	d	d	d
Comorbidity = 0.00	−0.204	−0.204	−0.339	−1.359	0.951
Comorbidity = 1.00	d	d	d	d	d

[a]Dependent variable: effect treatment
[b]Model: (intercept), group, male/female, comorbidity
[c]Assume standard reference priors
[d]This parameter Is redundant. Posterior statistics are not calculated.

Bayesian estimates of error variane[a]

Parameter	Posterior			95% Credible interval	
	Mode	Mean	Variance	Lower bound	Upper bound
Error variance	1.099	1.412	0.332	0.686	2.863

[a]Assume standard reference priors

The ANOVA table is identical to the one of the traditional multiple regression. The second table gives the Bayes factor of the analysis data model. The Bayes factor of this multiple model is much smaller than it is with the simple linear regression model (1.626 versus 17.329), meaning here less support against the null hypothesis and in favor of the alternative hypothesis. The third table gives posterior Bayesian regression coefficients of the predictor variables versus regression coefficients of zero. The maximal likelihoods of the predictors are given. They are at the same time the modes and means of the variables. It is interesting to observe that, although their 95% confidence intervals (to avoid confusion here named credible intervals) are approximately equal, $\approx$2.2–2.3, their modes and means are very different, 1.642, 0.390, −0.204. As explained in the Chap.1 this means that the area under the curve of the likelihood distribution of wide interval predictors are much larger than they are with small interval predictors. Obviously the small interval predictor, the groups variable, gives a lot more predictive certainty than the other two do.

The Bayes factor (BF) in this example of 1.626 is only slightly >1.0 and compatible with the p-value of 0.021 (as obtained from the traditional linear regression), which is also only slightly smaller than <0.05.

On a continuous line of Bayes factors from >30 to 1.0, our Bayes factor is not far from the right side end of BF = 1.0.

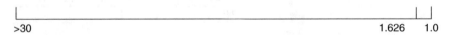

>30   1.626   1.0

On a continuous line of p-values from 0.0 to 0.05 our p-value is again not far from the right end side.

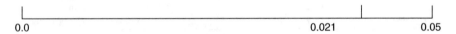

0.0   0.021   0.05

The above Bayes factor table shows that a Bayes factor of >1 supports the alternative hypothesis, an overall statistically significant multiple regression model. The BF of 1.626, thus, supports that of the traditional regression. In conclusion, a Bayes factor of 1.626 gives support in favor of the alternative hypothesis and against the null hypothesis.

7.7   Traditional Linear Regression Analysis with a Continuous Predictor

A Bayesian linear regression with a continuous predictor rather than binary is possible in SPSS. However, the continuous variable must be entered as covariate. The above example will be used again, but, instead of group as binary independent variable, age as continuous variable will be entered.

Commands:
as given above.
The output sheets are given below.

Variables entered/removed[a]

Model	Variables entered	Variables removed	Method
1	Age[b]		Enter

[a]Dependent variable: effect treatment
[b]All requested variables entered

Model summary

Model	R	R square	Adjusted R square	Std. error of the estimate
1	0.975[a]	0.950	0.947	0.31626

[a]Predictors: (constant), age

ANOVA[a]

Model		Sum of squares	df	Mean square F	F	Sig.
1	Regression	34,022	1	34,022	340.156	0.000[b]
	Residual	1,800	18	,100		
	Total	35,822	19			

[a]Dependent variable: effect treatment
[b]Predictors: (constant), age

Coefficients[a]

Model		Unstandardized coefficients		Standardized coefficients		
		B	Std. error	Beta	t	Sig.
1	(Constant)	0.282	0.322		0.877	0.392
	Age	0.093	0.005	0.975	18.443	0.000

[a]Dependent variable: effect treatment

The traditional linear regression with a single continuous predictor is above. Age is a very significant predictor of the outcome hours of sleep. The Bayesian linear regression with as covariate a single continuous predictor, age, is underneath.

7.8   Bayesian Linear Regression Analysis with a Continuous Predictor

Commands:
as given above.
The output sheets are given below.

ANOVA[a,b]

Source	Sum of squares	df	Mean square	F	Sig.
Regression	34,022	1	34,022	340.156	0.000

Source	Sum of squares	df	Mean square	F	Sig.
Residual	1,800	18	,100		
Total	35,822	19			

[a]Dependent variable: effect treatment
[b]Model: (intercept), age

Bayes factor model summary[a,b]

Bayes factor[c]	R	R square	Adjusted R square	Std. error of the estimate
2.284E + 10	0.975	0.950	0.947	0.3163

[a]Method: JZS
[b]Model: (intercept), age
[c]Bayes factor: testing model versus null model (Intercept)

Bayesian estimates of coefficients[a,b,c]

Parameter	Posterior			95% Credible interval	
	Mode	Mean	Variance	Lower bound	Upper bound
(Intercept)	0.282	0.282	0.116	−0.394	0.958
Age	0.093	0.093	0.000	0.082	0.104

[a]Dependent variable: effect treatment
[b]Model: (intercept), age
[c]Assume standard reference priors

Bayesian estimates of error variance[a]

Parameter	Posterior			95% Credible interval	
	Mode	Mean	Variance	Lower bound	Upper bound
Error variance	0.090	0.113	0.002	0.057	0.219

[a]Assume standard reference priors

The first table gives the analysis of variance of the predictor age versus the outcome hours of sleep. Age obviously determines hours of sleep at $p < 0.0001$. The second table gives the BF which is huge, 2.284^{10}. Extreme support is given for H1. The third table shows that the 95% credible interval of the likelihood distribution with maximal likelihood of 0.093 is very small, namely $0.104 - 0.082 = 0.022$. This means much certainty is given by the predictor age.

The Bayes factor (BF) in this example of 2.284^{10} giving very strong support of the alternative hypothesis, is compatible with the p-value of <0.0001 (as obtained from the traditional linear regression).

On a continuous line of Bayes factors from >30 to 1.0, our Bayes factor is very much skewed to the left end side.

⌐|——————————————————————————————|
>30 2.284^{10} 1.0

On a continuous line of p-values from 0.0 to 0.05 our p-value is again very much skewed to the left end side.

```
|_|_____|
0.0    <0.0001                                          0.05
```

The above Bayes factor table shows that a Bayes factor of 2.284^{10} very much supports the alternative hypothesis, a significant regression model with a continuous predictor. This result, thus, supports that of the traditional regression. And so, this Bayes factor gives support in favor of the alternative hypothesis and against the null hypothesis.

7.9 Conclusion

Bayesian regression analysis uses credible intervals and Bayes factor (BF) to predict the support of a null (H0) and alternative hypothesis (H1). Usually credible intervals are wider than 95% confidence intervals, but with regressions these intervals are largely similar. Unlike with Bayesian one sample tests and t-tests, with Bayesian regressions BFs are not computed with support of H0 versus H1, but, in contrast, the other way around. This may be convenient, because regressions are usually explorative and multiple BFs need to be compared in order to find the best fit models. However, it is no necessity. Advantages of the Bayesian approach may include.

1. A better underlying structure of the H1 and H0 may be provided.
2. Bayesian tests work with 95% credible intervals that are usually somewhat wider and this may reduce the chance of statistical significances with little clinical relevance.
3. Maximal likelihoods of likelihood distributions are not always identical to the mean effect of traditional tests, and this may be fine, because biological likelihoods may better fit biological questions than numerical means of non-representative subgroups do.
4. Bayes uses ratios of likelihood distributions rather than ratios of Gaussian distributions, which are notorious for ill data fit.
5. Bayesian integral computations are very advanced, and, therefore, give optimal precisions of complex functions, and better so than traditional multiple mean calculations of non representative subsamples do.
6. With Bayesian testing type I and II errors need not being taken into account.

A disadvantage of Bayesian analysis is an increased risk of overfitting, but in the regression examples of this chapter this was virtually not observed.

Suggested Reading[1,2]

Statistics applied to clinical studies 5th edition, 2012
Machine learning in medicine a complete overview, 2015
SPSS for starters and 2nd levelers 2nd edition, 2015
Clinical data analysis on a pocket calculator 2nd edition, 2016
Understanding clinical data analysis from published research, 2016
Modern Meta-analysis, 2017, Regression Analysis in Clinical Research, 2018

---

[1] To readers requesting more background, theoretical and mathematical information of computations given, several textbooks complementary to the current production and written by the same authors are available.

[2] All of them have been written by the same authors, and they have been edited by Springer Heidelberg Germany.

Chapter 8
Bayesian Analysis of Variance (Anova)

8.1 Background

In studies with two unpaired samples of continuous data as outcome and a binary predictor like treatment modality unpaired t-tests are usually applied. With three or more unpaired samples traditional t-tests are impossible, and analysis of variance (anova) must be applied. The mean values per group are squared and after adjustment for degrees of freedom divided by the squared standard deviations of the groups. The division sum, called the F (Fisher)-statistic, should be larger than approximately "5 or so" in order for the null hypothesis of no difference between variability of the treatment groups to be rejected, as tested against the variability of the subjects (within the groups). Instead of a traditional Anova a Bayesian Anova is possible. It assesses the magnitude the Bayes factor (BF) as computed from the ratio of a posterior and prior likelihood distribution. The posterior is modeled from the means and variances of the measured unpaired groups, the prior is usually modeled as an uninformative prior either from the Jeffreys Zellner Siow (JZS) method or, equivalently, from the computation of a reference prior based on a gamma distribution with a standard error of "1". The computation of the BF requires integral calculations for accuracy purposes. But, then, it can be used as a statistical index that pretty precisely quantifies the amount of support in favor of either H1 (the difference between the unpaired means is larger than zero) or H0 (the difference between the unpaired means is not larger than zero). Advantages of the Bayesian approach may include.

1. A better underlying structure model of the H1 and H0 may be provided.
2. Maximal likelihoods of likelihood distributions are not always identical to the mean effect of traditional tests, and this may be fine, because biological likelihoods may better fit biological questions than numerical means of non-representative subgroups do.

© Springer International Publishing AG, part of Springer Nature 2018
T. J. Cleophas, A. H. Zwinderman, *Modern Bayesian Statistics in Clinical Research*,
https://doi.org/10.1007/978-3-319-92747-3_8

However, in spite of this, nobody knows for sure why likelihood distributions may better than normal distributions estimate uncertainties in statistical test results. So, why not use both methods for analyzing the same data example. The current chapter will show and compare the results of traditional anova with that of Bayesian anova.

For convenience a data file is in extras.springer.com, and is entitled "chap8".

8.2   Data Example

The data file is opened in your computer with SPSS statistical software version 25 loaded including the module advanced statistics. A 30 patient parallel group study with three treatment modalities is used to answer the scientific question: do two sleeping pills and a placebo produce significantly different magnitudes of numbers of sleeping hours.

Variable				
1	2	3	4	5
0,00	6,00	45,00	0,00	1,00
0,00	7,10	45,00	0,00	1,00
0,00	8,10	46,00	0,00	0,00
0,00	7,50	37,00	0,00	0,00
0,00	6,40	48,00	0,00	1,00
0,00	7,90	76,00	1,00	1,00
0,00	6,80	56,00	1,00	1,00
0,00	6,60	54,00	1,00	0,00
0,00	7,30	63,00	1,00	0,00
0,00	5,60	75,00	0,00	0,00
1,00	5,10	64,00	1,00	0,00
1,00	8,00	35,00	0,00	1,00
1,00	3,80	46,00	1,00	0,00
1,00	4,40	44,00	0,00	1,00
1,00	5,20	64,00	1,00	0,00
1,00	5,40	75,00	0,00	1,00
1,00	4,30	65,00	1,00	1,00
1,00	6,00	84,00	1,00	0,00
1,00	3,70	35,00	1,00	0,00
1,00	6,20	46,00	0,00	1,00
2,00	4,10	43,00	0,00	0,00
2,00	7,00	56,00	0,00	0,00
2,00	2,80	65,00	0,00	0,00
2,00	3,40	66,00	0,00	1,00
2,00	4,20	74,00	1,00	1,00
2,00	4,40	56,00	1,00	1,00
2,00	3,30	45,00	0,00	1,00

Variable				
1	2	3	4	5
2,00	5,00	47,00	1,00	1,00
2,00	2,70	65,00	0,00	1,00
2,00	5,20	56,00	1,00	0,00

Variable 1 = group 0 has placebo, group 1 has sleeping pill 1, group 2 sleeping pill 2
Variable 2 = hours of sleep
Variable 3 = age
Variable 4 = gender
Variable 5 = co-morbidity

In the above table are the data of a parallel group study of three groups assessed for hours of sleep after treatment with a placebo or one of two sleeping pills. With three treatment modalities t-tests can not be used for an overall comparison. Analysis of variance must be used to test the null hypothesis that the treatments are equal. First, a traditional and then a Bayesian anova will be performed.

8.3   Traditional Analysis of Variance (Anova)

Start by opening the data file in your computer mounted with SPSS (version 25) statistical software module Bayesian statistics.

Command:
Analyze....Compare Means....One-Way Anova....Dependent List: effect treatment....
   Factor: group....click OK.

Descriptives
Effect treatment

					95% Confidence interval for mean			
	N	Mean	Std. deviation	Std. error	Lower bound	Upper bound 1	Minimum 1	Maximum
0.00	10	6.9300	0.80561	0.25475	6.3537	7.5063	5.60	8.10
1.00	10	5.2100	1.29910	0.41081	4.2807	6.1393	3.70	8.00
2.00	10	4.2100	1.29910	0.41081	3.2807	5.1393	2.70	7.00
Total	30	5.4500	1.59822	0.29179	4.8532	6.0468	2.70	8.10

ANOVA
Effect treatment

	Sum of squares	df	Mean square	F	Sig.
Between groups	37,856	2	18,928	14.110	0.000
Within groups	36,219	27	1,341		
Total	74,075	29			

The two tables in the output sheets are above. The ANOVA table shows that the differences between the groups is significantly larger than the differences between the subjects, and the null hypothesis (H0) of no difference between between-group and within group is rejected at p < 0.0001. This does not imply that that the alternative hypothesis H1 (the presence of a real difference in the data) is true because this was not assessed. The above first table gives descriptives, and it can be observed that the 95% confidence interval of the group zero does not overlap the 95% confidence intervals of the groups 1 and 2, and so this would mean that the average of sleeping hours in the Group 0 is significantly different from both the group 2 and 3 mean hours of sleep. The Bayesian approach is different. It should show whether the likelihood distributions of H1 and H0 and their ratio support H1 or not.

8.4   Bayesian Analysis of Variance (Anova)

Note:
One way Anova is a bit like linear regression. It has dependent and independent variables. Regressions and Anovas are usually explorative, and multiple models are compared for best fit prediction. Bayes factors are used for comparing the results. Large Bayes factors (BFs) may be more convenient for explorative purposes than small ones. Like with linear regression (Chap. 9), Bayes is here not computed with "supporting null versus alternative hypothesis" but, in contrast, the other way around. This would mean that, with a large Bayes factor (BF), H1 is strongly supported, and, thus, H0 is not so.

Command:
Analyze....Bayesian Statistics....One-way Anova....Dependent: effect treatment....Factor:group....Bayes Analysis: mark Use Both Methods....click Criteria: default settings....click Continue....click Priors: click Reference priors, otherwise default settings....click Continue....click OK.

The underneath tables are in the output.

ANOVA

Effect treatment	Sum of squares	df	Mean square	F	Sig.	Bayes factor[a]
Between groups	37,856	2	18,928	14.110	0.000	389.479
Within groups	36,219	27	1,341			
Total	74,075	29				

[a]Bayes factor: JZS

Bayesian estimates of coefficients[a,b,c]

	Posterior			95% Credible interval	
Parameter	Mode	Mean	Variance	Lower bound	Upper bound
Group = 0.00	6.930	6.930	0.145	6.179	7.681

| Group = 1.00 | 5.210 | 5.210 | 0.145 | 4.459 | 5.961 |
| Group = 2.00 | 4.210 | 4.210 | 0.145 | 3.459 | 4.961 |

[a]Dependent variable: effect treatment
[b]Model: group
[c]Assume standard reference priors

Bayesian estimates of error variance[a]

Parameter	Mode	Posterior Mean	Variance	95% Credible interval Lower bound	Upper bound
Error variance	1.249	1.449	0.183	0.839	2.485

[a]Assume standard reference priors

The first table is largely similar to the traditional anova table. The footnote mentions the use of a JZS (Jeffrey Zellner Siow) method. It is a way for computing priors equivalent to those computed with standard beta (for binomial data) and gamma (for continuous and normal data) distributions with a standard error of 1. It is usually named together with reference priors because of their references to the standard data distributions. These priors are adequate for Bayesian linear regressions and Bayesian analyses of variance. The computed BF equals 389.479, and according to the underneath scheme it follows that we have extreme support for the alternative hypothesis.

Reject H0

Bayes Factor	Evidence Category	Bayes Factor	Evidence Category	Bayes Factor	Evidence Category
>100	Extreme Evidence for H1	1-3	Anecdotal Evidence for H1	1/30-1/10	Strong Evidence for H0
30-100	Very Strong Evidence for H1	1	No Evidence	1/100-1/30	Very Strong Evidence for H0
10-30	Strong Evidence for H1	1/3-1	Anecdotal Evidence for H0	1/100	Extreme Evidence for H0
3-10	Moderate Evidence for H1	1/10-1/3	Moderate Evidence for H0		

Reject H1

The third above table gives the Bayesian estimates of coefficients. It is comparable with the descriptive data from the traditional ANOVA output, but, instead of means and standard errors and 95% confidence intervals, 95% credible intervals from likelihood distributions, are given. The means and modes are identical, and are at the same time maximal likelihoods. The 95% credible intervals give an impression about the widths of the likelihood distributions:

	95% confidence interval	95% credible interval
Group 0.0	6.3537–7.5063	6.179–7.681
Group 1.0	4.2807–6.1393	4.459–5.961
Group 3.0	3.2807–5.1393	3.459–4.961

The group 0 credible interval is a bit wider than the traditional 95% confidence interval is. The groups 2 and 3 credible intervals are a bit narrower. Obviously, group 0 provides the best likelihood in favor of H1.

The Bayes factor (BF) in this example of 389.479 gives very strong support of the alternative hypothesis, and is compatible with the p-value of <0.0001 (as obtained from the traditional linear anova).

On a continuous line of Bayes factors from >30 to 1.0, our Bayes factor is very much skewed to the left end side.

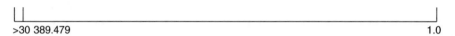

>30 389.479   1.0

On a continuous line of p-values from 0.0 to 0.05 our p-value is equally very much skewed to the left end side.

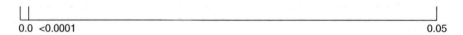

0.0 <0.0001   0.05

The above Bayes factor table shows that a Bayes factor of 389.479 very much supports the alternative hypothesis, a statistically significant anova model. This result, thus, supports that of the traditional anova. And so, this Bayes factor gives support in favor of the alternative hypothesis and against the null hypothesis.

8.5   Conclusion

This chapter assesses the performance of Bayesian anova as compared to traditional anova. Generally, Bayesian estimators were very well compatible with traditional test estimators.

Advantages of the Bayesian approach may include.

1. A better underlying structure of the H1 and H0 may be provided.
2. Bayesian tests work with 95% credible intervals that are usually somewhat wider and this may reduce the chance of statistical significances with little clinical relevance.
3. maximal likelihoods of likelihood distributions are not always identical to the mean effect of traditional tests, and this may be fine, because biological likelihoods may better fit biological questions than numerical means of non-representative subgroups do.

4. Bayes uses ratios of likelihood distributions rather than ratios of Gaussian distributions, which are notorious for ill data fit.
5. Bayesian integral computations are very advanced, and, therefore, give optimal precisions of complex functions, and better so than traditional multiple mean calculations of non representative subsamples do.
6. With Bayesian testing type I and II errors need not being taken into account.

A disadvantage of Bayesian analysis may be an increased risk of overfitting: the likelihood distribution and the ratio of likelihood distributions of the Bayesian analyses may be wider than compatible with Gaussian modeling. For example, the 95% credible interval of group 0 is between 6.179 and 7.681. The 95% confidence interval of the mean and 95% Gaussian confidence interval is between 6.354 and 7.506 which is narrower an interval than 95% credible interval is.

With Bayes factors (BFs) sometimes but not always a better test statistic of your data is provided, but not always. In this chapter both the BF (389.479) and the p-value (p < 0.0001) provided extreme support of the alternative hypothesis H1.

Suggested Reading[1,2]

Statistics applied to clinical studies 5th edition, 2012
Machine learning in medicine a complete overview, 2015
SPSS for starters and 2nd levelers 2nd edition, 2015
Clinical data analysis on a pocket calculator 2nd edition, 2016
Understanding clinical data analysis from published research, 2016
Modern Meta-analysis, 2017
Regression Analysis in Clinical Research, 2018

---

[1] To readers requesting more background, theoretical and mathematical information of computations given, several textbooks complementary to the current production and written by the same authors are available.

[2] All of them have been written by the same authors and they have been edited by Springer Heidelberg Germany.

Chapter 9
Bayesian Loglinear Regression

9.1 Background

In studies with both a binary outcome (for example event yes/no) and binary predictor variable (for example treatment group 1 or 2) for traditional analysis a 2 × 2 interaction matrix is drawn with the predictor in two rows and the outcome in two columns. The null hypothesis H0 is defined as "no difference between the treatment groups", the alternative hypothesis H1 is defined as "a real difference between the treatment groups". Usually the chi-square test is applied for assessing whether the null hypothesis of no difference between the two groups can be rejected. If not, the alternative hypothesis can not be accepted because this was not assessed. Instead of a 2 × 2 chi-square test also a Bayesian loglinear regression is possible. It assesses the magnitude of the Bayes factor (BF). A BF smaller than "one" supports the above alternative hypothesis (H1), while a BF larger than "one" supports the above null hypothesis (H0). The BF is computed as the ratio of two likelihood distributions, that of the posterior and the prior likelihood distribution. The posterior is modeled from the measured proportions of patients with an event, the prior is modeled with the help of a conjugate prior, which is a way for computing a prior the same as that of the measured posterior likelihood distribution, however, with a standard error of "1".

The computation of the BF requires integrations for accuracy purposes. But, then, it can be used as a statistical index to pretty precisely quantify the amount of support in favor H1 and H0. Advantages of the Bayesian approach may include.

1. A better underlying structure model of the H1 and H0 may be provided.
2. Maximal likelihoods of likelihood distributions are not always identical to the mean effect of traditional tests, and this may be fine, because biological likelihoods may better fit biological questions than numerical means of non-representative subgroups do.

© Springer International Publishing AG, part of Springer Nature 2018

T. J. Cleophas, A. H. Zwinderman, *Modern Bayesian Statistics in Clinical Research*,
https://doi.org/10.1007/978-3-319-92747-3_9

However, in spite of this, nobody knows for sure why likelihood distributions may better than normal distributions estimate uncertainties in statistical test results. So, why not use both of them for analyzing the same data example. The current chapter will show and compare the results of traditional 2 × 2 chi-square-tests and the Bayesian loglinear regression for 2 × 2 interaction matrices. For self-assessment a data file is in extras.springer.com, and is entitled "chap9".

9.2   Introduction

The underneath table are the data of a study of 30 patients admitted to two hospital departments, surgery and internal medicine. The primary scientific question was: is there a significant difference between the risks of falling out of bed at the departments of surgery and internal medicine.

	Fall out of bed	
	No	Yes
Number of patient department surgery (0)	20	15
Internal department (1)	5	15

The above interaction matrix of the data shows that at both departments the same numbers of patients fall out of bed. However, at the department of surgery many more patients do not fall out of bed than at the internal department.

Variable

1	2	3	4	5
,00	1,00	60,00	,00	1,00
,00	1,00	86,00	,00	1,00
,00	1,00	67,00	1,00	1,00
,00	1,00	75,00	,00	1,00
,00	1,00	56,00	1,00	1,00
,00	1,00	46,00	1,00	1,00
,00	1,00	98,00	,00	,00
,00	1,00	66,00	1,00	,00
,00	1,00	54,00	,00	,00
,00	1,00	86,00	1,00	1,00
,00	1,00	86,00	1,00	1,00
,00	1,00	84,00	1,00	1,00
,00	1,00	87,00	,00	,00
,00	1,00	55,00	,00	,00
,00	1,00	56,00	1,00	,00
,00	,00	37,00	,00	,00
,00	,00	38,00	1,00	,00
,00	,00	77,00	,00	,00

| Variable | | | | |
1	2	3	4	5
,00	,00	55,00	,00	,00
,00	,00	40,00	1,00	,00
,00	,00	39,00	,00	,00
,00	,00	48,00	1,00	1,00
,00	,00	83,00	,00	,00
,00	,00	74,00	1,00	1,00
,00	,00	47,00	1,00	1,00
,00	,00	38,00	,00	,00
,00	,00	25,00	,00	,00
,00	,00	16,00	1,00	,00
,00	,00	66,00	1,00	,00
,00	,00	46,00	,00	,00
,00	,00	46,00	,00	,00
,00	,00	25,00	1,00	,00
,00	,00	19,00	,00	,00
,00	,00	68,00	,00	,00
,00	,00	57,00	,00	,00
1,00	1,00	64,00	1,00	,00
1,00	1,00	75,00	1,00	,00
1,00	1,00	84,00	1,00	1,00
1,00	1,00	83,00	,00	1,00
1,00	1,00	95,00	,00	1,00
1,00	1,00	75,00	,00	1,00
1,00	1,00	84,00	1,00	1,00
1,00	1,00	75,00	1,00	1,00
1,00	1,00	85,00	1,00	1,00
1,00	1,00	65,00	,00	1,00
1,00	1,00	74,00	1,00	1,00
1,00	1,00	87,00	,00	,00
1,00	1,00	76,00	1,00	,00
1,00	1,00	96,00	,00	,00
1,00	1,00	86,00	1,00	,00
1,00	,00	45,00	,00	,00
1,00	,00	56,00	1,00	,00
1,00	,00	57,00	,00	,00
1,00	,00	56,00	1,00	,00
1,00	,00	48,00	,00	1,00

Var 1 = department (0 = department surgery, 1 = internal department) (Var = variable)
Var 2 = falling out of bed (1 = yes, 0 = no)
Var 3 = age
Var 4 = gender
Var 5 = letter of complaint (1 = yes, 0 = no).

9.3   Traditional Chi-Square Analysis for 2 × 2 Interaction Matrix

The data file stored at extras.springer.com and entitled "chap9" will first be used for drawing a three dimensional graph of the data. Open the data in SPSS statistical software version 25 (with the Advanced Statistics module included) by clicking the title in your computer mounted with SPSS. Then command.

Command:
click Graphs....click 3D Charts....X-Axis: enter departments....Z-Axis: enter falling out of bed....click OK.

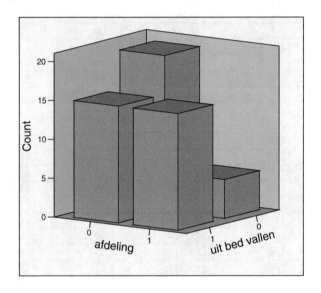

At both departments approximately the same number of patients fall out of bed. However, at department-0 many more patients do not fall out of bed than at department-1 do.

9.4   Traditional Analysis for 2 × 2 Interaction Matrix: The Chi-Square Test

Command:
Analyze....Descriptive   Statistics....Crosstabs....Rows: enter   variable   1.... Columns: enter variable 2....Statistics....Chi-Square....click OK.

The table below is in the SPSS output sheets.

Chi-square tests

	Value	df	Asy mp. sig. (2-sided)	Exact sig. (2-sided)	Exact sig. (1-sided)
Pearson chi-square	5.304[a]	1	0.021		
Continuity correction	4.086	1	0.043		
Likelihood ratio	5.494	1	0.019		
Fisher's exact test				0.027	0.021
Linear-by-linear association	5.207	1	0.022		
N of valid cases	55				

[a]0 cells (0.0%) have expected count less than 5. The minimum expected count is 9.09

The chi-square test (Pearson Chi-Square) shows, that a significant difference between the surgical and internal departments exists in patterns of patients falling out of bed. The p-value equals 0.021, and this is much smaller than 0.05. Several contrast tests have been given in the above results table. They produce approximately similar p-values. This supports the accuracy of the chi-square test for these data.

We have cells with only five counts, and, so, the traditional chi-square is flawed. We can nonetheless conclude that the null hypothesis of no difference between the two departments can be rejected. We can not conclude from this, that the alternative hypothesis, a true difference between the two departments, is true, because this was not assessed. In order to better assess the real meaning of our data result, and answer the question what level of likelihood we have to support either the null (H0) or the alternative hypothesis (H1), a modern Bayesian linear regression analysis will be performed. For that purpose in SPSS statistical software module v 25 a Bayesian loglinear regression analysis will be performed.

9.5 Bayesian Loglinear Regression for 2 × 2 Interaction Matrix

Command:
Analyze...Bayesian Statistics....Loglinear Models....Row variable: enter department ....Column variable: enter outcome....Bayesian Analysis: mark Use Both Methods....click Criteria: leave default setting....click Continue....click Bayes Factor: mark Conjugate, otherwise default setting....click Continue....click OK.

The four tables below are in the output sheets.

Case processing summary

	Valid		Missing		Total	
Observed cases	N	Percent	N	Percent	N	Percent
Department* outcome	55	90.2%	6	9.8%	61	100.0%

Department * outcome category tabulation

			outcome		
			0.00	1.00	Total
department	0.00	Count	20	15	35
	1.00	Count	5	15	20
Total		Count	25	30	55

Test of independence[a]

	Value	df	Asymptotic sig. (2-sided)	Exact sig. (2-sided)	Exact sig. (1-sided)
Bayes factor	0.161[b]				
Pearson chi-square	5.304[c]	1	0.021		
Continuity correction	4.086	1	0.043		
Fisher's exact test				0.027	0.021

[a]The total sum is fixed in the contingencytable
[b]This analysis tests independence versus association, and assumes a multinomial model and conjugate priors
[c]0 cells(0.0%) have expected count less than 5. The minimum expected count is 9.091

Posterior distribution characterization of simulated interactions[a,b]

	Posterior			95% Simultaneous credible interval		
Interaction	Median	Mean	Variance	Lower bound	Upper bound	Contains 0 or not
0.00, 0.00	1.301	1.314	0.359	0.176	2.528	No

[a]The analyses assume an independent multinomial model
[b]Seed: 599767049. Number ofsimulated posterior samples: 1,000,000

The first and second Bayesian tables give simply summary statistics. The third table reports the tests of independence versus association, or support for real difference between the departments or not. In addition to the test statistics similar to those of the traditional chi-square tests, the Bayes factor (BF) is given. It is computed from the division sum of posterior and prior likelihood distributions where posterior and prior are based on respectively the observed data and, in the absence of an informed prior, a conjugate measure obtained from the posterior, however with a standard error of 1. The above fourth table gives the statistics of the posterior. Footnote c shows that Monte Carlo simulations were applied to integrate out the nuisance parameter, a parameter not directly of interest to the ratio of likelihood distributions. After many iterations it is zero. The median and mean of the selected posterior distribution are not normal and slightly skewed to the right.

Nonetheless it performed well enough, and the ratio of posterior and prior, the Bayes factor, was pretty small, 0.161. This indicates that we have moderate to strong support for the alternative hypothesis, a real difference between the two departments. This result is in agreement with the above results from the traditional chi-square test.

The underneath Bayes factor table given by SPSS is helpful here.

Reject H1

Bayes Factor	Evidence Category	Bayes Factor	Evidence Category	Bayes Factor	Evidence Category
>100	Extreme Evidence for H0	1-3	Anecdotal Evidence for H0	1/30-1/10	Strong Evidence for H1
30-100	Very Strong Evidence for H0	1	No Evidence	1/100-1/30	Very Strong Evidence for H1
10-30	Strong Evidence for H0	1/3-1	Anecdotal Evidence for H1	1/100	Extreme Evidence for H1
3-10	Moderate Evidence for H0	1/10-/1-/3	Moderate Evidence for H1		

Reject H0

Bayesian loglinear also produces statistics of counts observed and expected. For the computation the default command is: first click Print. Then mark Expected Counts, Percentages Row, Column, and Total. The underneath table is in the SPSS output.

Department * outcome category tabulation

			outcome		
			0.00	1.00	Total
department	0.00	Count	20	15	35
		Expected count	15.9	19.1	35.0
		% within department	57.1%	42.9%	100.0%
		% within outcome	80.0%	50.0%	63.6%
		% of total	36.4%	27.3%	63.6%
	1.00	Count	5	15	20
		Expected count	9.1	10.9	20.0
		% within department	25.0%	75.0%	100.0%
		% within outcome	20.0%	50.0%	36.4%
		% of total	9.1%	27.3%	36.4%
Total		Count	25	30	55
		Expected count	25.0	30.0	55.0
		% within department	45.5%	54.5%	100.0%
		% within outcome	100.0%	100.0%	100.0%
		% of total	45.5%	54.5%	100.0%

Obviously, the departments (0) and (1) are analyzed separately: the proportions "fall out of bed" "yes" or "no" per department are reported both separately and together.

9.6 Conclusion

This chapter assesses Bayesian loglinear regression and Bayesian interaction matrix analysis. The Bayesian approach pretty much matches traditional analysis methods.

With modern Bayesian statistics likelihood distributions rather than probability distributions are modeled. It is mostly based on the Cauchy distribution, a member of the family of the alpha distributions, and the distribution that best describes the ratio of either two normal distributions or two likelihood distributions. Bayes factors have a Cauchy distribution, and cannot be numerically analyzed with standard Gaussian approximation methods. Fortunately, pretty good numerical results are obtained by integrations that integrate out nuisance variables.

Advantages of the Bayesian approach may include.

1. A better underlying structure of the H1 and H0 may be provided.
2. Bayesian tests work with 95% credible intervals that are usually somewhat wider and this may reduce the chance of statistical significances with little clinical relevance.
3. Maximal likelihoods of likelihood distributions are not always identical to the mean effect of traditional tests, and this may be fine, because biological likelihoods may better fit biological questions than numerical means of non-representative subgroups do.
4. Bayes uses ratios of likelihood distributions rather than ratios of Gaussian distributions, which are notorious for ill data fit.
5. Bayesian integral computations are very advanced, and, therefore, give optimal precisions of complex functions, and better so than traditional multiple mean calculations of non representative subsamples do.
6. With Bayesian testing type I and II errors need not being taken into account.

A disadvantage of Bayesian methods may be overfitting. This means that the likelihood distributions may be wider than compatible Gaussian modeling. Bootstraps t-test is based on Monte Carlo resampling from your own data. It is available in SPSS statistical software. In the example given we will compare a bootstraps sampling distribution in SPSS with Bayesian likelihood and traditional Gaussian distributions. Once again the data example from the current chapter is used.

Command:
Analyze....Regression....Binary Logistic Regression....Dependent: fall out of bed....Covariate(s) Department....click Bootstrap....click Perform bootstrapping....Number Samples enter 1000....click Continue....click OK.

The bootstrap resampling model is in the output sheets. It provides a 95% confidence interval between 0.176 and 3.043.

The Bayesian and traditional chi-square 95% confidence intervals are given above.

1. Gaussian 95% confidence interval 0.148 and 2.624
2. Bootstrap 95% confidence interval 0.176 and 3.043
3. Bayesian 95% credible interval 0.176 and 2.528.

Obviously, the Gaussian confidence interval, the bootstrap confidence interval, and the Bayesian credible interval have very much similarly sized intervals. Overfitting is not obvious.

The Bayes factor (BF) in this chapter's example of 0.161 suggests that the Bayesian one sample t-test model provides a better sensitivity of testing than the traditional one sample continuous data t-test model does.

On a continuous line of Bayes factors from 1.0 to 0.0 our Bayes factor is on the right side.

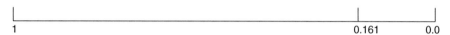

On a continuous line of p-values from 0.05 to 0.0 our p-value is closer to the middle.

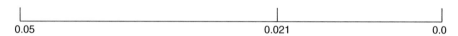

The BF of 0.161 is closer to 0.0 (or very small), than the p-value of 0.021 is. The BF seems to provide a slightly better statistic here than the p-value does.

Suggested Reading[1,2]

Statistics applied to clinical studies 5th edition, 2012
Machine learning in medicine a complete overview, 2015
SPSS for starters and 2nd levelers 2nd edition, 2015
Clinical data analysis on a pocket calculator 2nd edition, 2016
Understanding clinical data analysis from published research, 2016
Modern Meta-analysis, 2017
Regression Analysis in Clinical Research, 2018

[1] To readers requesting more background, theoretical and mathematical information of computations given, several textbooks complementary to the current production and written by the same authors are available.

[2] All of them have been written by the same authors, and have been edited by Springer Heidelberg Germany.

Chapter 10
Bayesian Poisson Rate Analysis

10.1 Background

Poisson analysis is adequate for studies where event rate per patient per period of exposure is used as main outcome. Unlike normal distributions, the Poisson distribution depends on just one parameter which is the mean number of events per person per period of time. Its standard error equals $\sqrt{\text{mean}}$. The Poisson rate test assesses whether the mean rate of events and its 95% confidence interval (the alternative hypothesis H1) is significantly different from a mean rate of zero and the same 95% confidence interval (the null hypothesis H0). Instead of a traditional Poisson rate test also a Bayesian Poison rate test one sample normal test is possible. It assesses the magnitude of the Bayes factor (BF). A BF smaller than "one" supports the above alternative hypothesis (H1), while a BF larger than "one" supports the above null hypothesis (H0). The BF is computed as the ratio of two likelihood distributions, that of the posterior and the prior likelihood distribution. The posterior is modeled from the mean rate of the measured data and its 95% credible interval, the prior is modeled as a conjugate (= custom) prior based on the same distribution as that of the posterior data but with a standard error of "1". However, an uninformative uniform prior with a likelihood of "one" in the same interval as that of the posterior is pretty much OK as well. The computation of BF requires integrations for accuracy purposes. But, then, it can be used as a statistical index for quantifying the amount of support in favor H1 and H0. Advantages of the Bayesian approach may include.

1. A better underlying structure model of the H1 and H0 may be provided.
2. Maximal likelihoods of likelihood distributions are not always identical to the mean effect of traditional tests, and this may be fine, because biological likelihoods may better fit biological questions than numerical means of non-representative subgroups do.

© Springer International Publishing AG, part of Springer Nature 2018   101
T. J. Cleophas, A. H. Zwinderman, *Modern Bayesian Statistics in Clinical Research*,
https://doi.org/10.1007/978-3-319-92747-3_10

However, in spite of this, nobody knows for sure why likelihood distributions may better than normal distributions estimate uncertainties in statistical test results. So, why not use both of them for analyzing the same data example. The current chapter will show and compare the results of traditional one sample t-tests and Bayesian one sample t-tests. For self-assessment purposes a data file is in extras.springer.com, and is entitled "chap10". Open the data file in your computer with SPSS version 25 the module advanced statistics included.

10.2   Introduction

The table below are the data of 50 patients assessed for rates of paroxysmal atrial fibrillations (pafs).

treat	psych	soc	paf
1	56,99	42,45	4
1	37,09	46,82	4
0	32,28	43,57	2
0	29,06	43,57	3
0	6,75	27,25	3
0	61,65	48,41	13
0	56,99	40,74	11
1	10,39	15,36	7
1	50,53	52,12	10
1	49,47	42,45	9
0	39,56	36,45	4
1	33,74	13,13	5
0	62,91	62,27	5
0	65,56	44,66	3
1	23,01	25,25	1
1	75,83	61,04	0
0	41,31	49,47	1
0	41,89	65,56	0
1	65,56	46,82	2
1	13,13	6,75	24
0	33,02	42,45	2
1	55,88	64,87	0
1	45,21	55,34	1
1	56,99	44,66	0
0	31,51	38,35	8
1	52,65	50,00	3
1	17,26	6,75	7
0	33,02	40,15	0
1	61,04	57,55	2

treat	psych	soc	paf
1	66,98	71,83	0
1	1,01	45,21	0
0	38,35	35,13	1
1	44,66	46,82	3
1	44,12	46,82	0
1	59,85	46,29	0
0	32,28	47,35	28
1	23,01	49,47	8
1	70,94	61,04	5
1	1,01	1,01	2
0	41,89	52,12	27
0	40,15	35,13	5
0	41,31	38,35	18
0	44,66	58,69	19
1	38,35	42,45	9
1	32,28	1,01	9
0	37,09	32,28	4
1	63,55	57,55	2
1	43,57	41,31	3
1	33,02	24,17	9
0	68,49	59,26	20

treat = treatment modality
psych = psychological score
soc = social score
paf = episodes of paroxysmal atrial fibrillations (PAF) per patient in one day of observation

A Poisson regression for outcome rates was performed in SPSS statistical software using the generalized linear models module and an intercept only model.

10.3   Traditional Generalized Linear Model Poisson-Analysis

Command:
Analyze….Generalized Linear Models….mark: Custom….Distribution: Poisson
…..Link function: Log….Response: Dependent variable: numbers of episodes of PAF….click Model: no predictor, intercept only model….click OK.

The underneath tables were in the output sheets

Model information

Dependent variable	Outcome rate
Probability distribution	Poisson
Link function	Log

Case processing summary

	N	Percent (%)
Included	50	100.0
Excluded	0	0.0
Total	50	100.0

Continuous variable information

	N	Minimum	Maximum	Mean	Std. deviation
Dependent variable: outcome rate	50	0	28	6.12	7.125

Omnibus test[a]

Likelihood ratio chi-square	df	Sig.
0.000		

Dependent variable: outcome rate
Model: (intercept)
[a]Compares the fitted model against the intercept-only model

Goodness of fit[a]

	Value	df	Value/df
Deviance	353.867	49	7.222
Scaled deviance	353.867	49	
Pearson chi-square	406.418	49	8.294
Scaled Pearson chi-square	406.418	49	
Log likelihood[b]	−248.362		
Akaike's information criterion (AIC)	498.725		
Finite sample corrected AIC (AICC)	498.808		
Bayesian information criterion (BIC)	500.637		
Consistent AIC (CAIC)	501.637		

Dependent variable: outcome rate
Model: (intercept)
[a]Information criteria are in smaller-is-betterform
[b]The full log likelihood function is displayed and used in computing information criteria

Tests of model effects

	Type III		
Source	Wald chi-square	df	Sig.
(Intercept)	1004.218	1	0.000

Dependent variable: outcome rate
Model: (intercept)

Parameter estimates

Parameter	B	Std. error	95% Wald confidence interval		Hypothesis test		
			Lower	Upper	Wald chi-square	df	Sig.
(Intercept)	1.812	0.0572	1.700	1.924	1004.218	1	0.000
(Scale)	1[a]						

Dependent variable: outcome rate
Model: (intercept)
[a]Fixed at the displayed value

The above continuous information criterion gives the mean rate per observation period of episodes of PAFs per patient. The goodness of fit table gives Akaike and Bayesian information criteria. They give like, just Bayesian factor analyses, likelihood functions that are approximately identically sized and have a largely similar meaning. These criteria are widely used within the world of traditional data analyses and observational data analyses. In itself these criteria do not mean too much, but applied in multiple variables models including additional variables they tend to fall. The lower the better fit of the models is obtained. This is however associated with increasing risk of model overfittings. The last two tables show that the null hypothesis of no difference from a rate of zero is rejected. A generalized linear regression model with rate of PAF per period of observation as outcome gives a p-value <0.0001. A Bayes factor analysis for Poisson rate testing will now be performed in order to assess whether support is established for the alternative hypothesis of a real difference from a likelihood of zero.

10.4   Bayesian Poisson Rate Analysis

Command:
Analyze....Bayesian Statistics....One Sample Poisson....Test Variable(s): enter paf....Bayes Analysis: Use Both Methods....Hypothesis Values: Alternate Prior Shape: enter 1...Alternate Prior Scale: enter 1....click Criteria: leave default setting....click Continue...click Priors: leave default setting....click Continue....click OK.

The underneath tables are in the output.

Bayes factor for Poisson Rate Test

	N	Counts		Bayes factor[a]
		Minimum	Maximum	
paf	50	0	28	0.061

[a]Bayes factor: null versus alternative hypothesis

Posterior distribution characterization for Poisson inference[a]

	Mode	Mean	Var.	95% Credible interval	
				Lower bound	Upper bound
outcome rate	5.90	5.92	0.114	5.28	6.60

[a]Prior for Poisson rate/Intensity; Gamma(2,2)

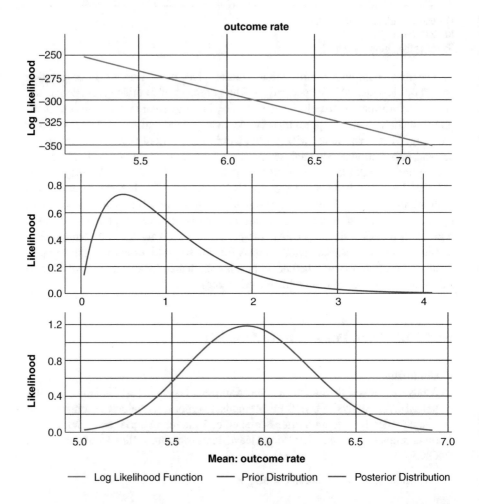

The Bayesian Poisson test assesses the division sum of posterior and prior likelihood distributions where posterior and prior are based on respectively the data given and either a gamma distribution suitable for binomials with nuisance parameters integrated out, or a conjugate prior with the same distribution as that of the posterior. The table shows, that its maximal likelihood is the mode of 5.9, which is slightly less than the mean score of 6.12 in the generalized linear model with a credible 95% interval 5.28—6.60. The 95% confidence interval of the traditional Poisson analysis is computed with logtransforms. The total numbers of PAFs = 306. The standard error (se) of the log of this total number is derived using the delta method (Cleophas and Zwinderman, Statistics applied to clinical studies 5th edition 2012, pp 524–525).

$$se\left(\log \text{total number}\right) = 1 / \sqrt{306} = 0.057$$

The 95% confidence interval of mean number can now be computed.

$$\log \text{ mean} \qquad = \log 6.12$$
$$= 1.812.$$

The log 95% confidence interval

$$= 1.812 \pm 2 \times 0.057$$
$$= \text{between } 1.698 \text{ and } 1.926.$$

The 95% confidence interval

$$= \text{antilog of log } 95\% \text{ confidence interval}$$
$$= \text{between } 5.463 \text{ and } 6.862$$
$$= 1.399.$$

This is hardly different from the above 95% credible interval of the

$$\text{Bayesian analysis} \qquad = \text{between } 5.28 \text{ and } 6.60$$
$$= 1.32.$$

The Bayes factor is computed 0.061. It is computed from the ratio of the posterior and prior likelihood distributions. For the latter of the two a conjugate (= custom) prior based on the same distribution as that of the posterior was used, but with a standard error of 1. The underneath scheme shows the relationships between Bayes factor magnitudes and support for either H0 or H1. Our Bayes factor of 0.061 indicates that H1 is strongly supported, which is in agreement with the above traditional analysis. This can be inferred from the underneath table from SPSS's help pages.

Bayes factor	Evidence category	Bayes factor	Evidence category	B ayes factor	Evidence category
>100	Extreme evidence for H0	1–3	Anecdotal evidence for H0	1/30 to 1/10	Strong evidence for H1
30–100	Very strong evidence for H0	1	No evidence	1/100 to 1/30	Very strong evidence for H1
10–30	Strong evidence for H0	1/3 to 1	Anecdotal evidence for H1	1/100	Extreme evidence for H1
3–10	Moderate evidence for H0	1/10 to 1/3	Moderate evidence for H1		

A slightly different and maybe helpful presentation of the above table we give underneath.

Reject H1

Bayes Factor	Evidence Category	Bayes Factor	Evidence Category	Bayes Factor	Evidence Category
>100	Extreme Evidence for H0	1-3	Anecdotal Evidence for H0	1/30-1/10	Strong Evidence for H1
30-100	Very Strong Evidence for H0	1	No Evidence	1/100-1/30	Very Strong Evidence for H1
10-30	Strong Evidence for H0	1/3-1	Anecdotal Evidence for H1	1/100	Extreme Evidence for H1
3-10	Moderate Evidence for H0	1/10/-1/3	Moderate Evidence for H1		

Reject H0

10.5   Conclusion

This chapter assesses Bayesian Poisson analysis. It performs generally equally well as does traditional Poisson analysis, although Bayesian statistics were generally slightly better sensitive.

With modern Bayesian statistics likelihood distributions are the main probability distribution model. It is mostly based on the Cauchy distribution, a member of the family of the alpha distributions, and the distribution that best describes the ratio of two normal distributions or two likelihood distributions. Bayes factors have a Cauchy distribution, and cannot be numerically analyzed with standard Gaussian approximation methods. Fortunately, pretty good numerical results are obtained by integrations that integrate out nuisance variables like noninformative priors or lacking priors. With rate data instead of normal distributions Poisson distributions are more adequate for data modeling than random normal data.

Advantages of the Bayesian approach may include.

1. A better underlying structure of the H1 and H0 may be provided.
2. Bayesian tests work with 95% credible intervals that are usually somewhat wider and this may reduce the chance of statistical significances with little clinical relevance.
3. Maximal likelihoods of likelihood distributions are not always identical to the mean effect of traditional tests, and this may be fine, because biological likelihoods may better fit biological questions than numerical means of non-representative subgroups do.
4. Bayes uses ratios of likelihood distributions rather than ratios of Gaussian distributions, which are notorious for ill data fit.
5. Bayesian integral computations are very advanced, and, therefore, give optimal precisions of complex functions, and better so than traditional multiple mean calculations of non representative subsamples do.
6. With Bayesian testing type I and II errors need not being taken into account.

A disadvantage of Bayesian methods may be overfitting. This means that the likelihood distributions may be wider than compatible Gaussian modeling. However, in the current example the Bayesian 95% credible interval and the 95% Poisson confidence interval were virtually identical.

The Bayes factor (BF) in this chapter's example of 0.506 suggests that the Bayesian one sample t-test model provides a slightly better sensitivity of testing than the traditional one sample continuous data t-test model does.

On a continuous line of Bayes factors from 1.0 to 0.0 our Bayes factor is very much on the right side.

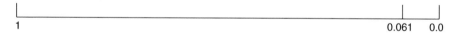

1   0.061   0.0

On a continuous line of p-values from 0.05 to 0.0 our p-value is similarly very much on the right side.

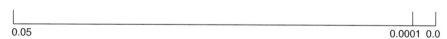

0.05   0.0001 0.0

The BF does not provide a better statistic here than does the p-value. The same was observed in the Chaps. 4–7. In contrast, a BF providing a better or compatible statistic than did the p-value was observed in the Chaps. 3, 8, and 9.

Suggested Reading[1,2]

Statistics applied to clinical studies 5th edition, 2012
Machine learning in medicine a complete overview, 2015
SPSS for starters and 2nd levelers 2nd edition, 2015
Clinical data analysis on a pocket calculator 2nd edition, 2016
Understanding clinical data analysis from published research, 2016
Modern Meta-analysis, 2017
Regression Analysis in Clinical Research, 2018

---

[1]To readers requesting more background, theoretical and mathematical information of computations given, several textbooks complementary to the current production and written by the same authors are available.

[2]All of them have been written by the same authors, and they have been edited by Springer Heidelberg Germany.

Chapter 11
Bayesian Pearson Correlation Analysis

11.1 Background

In studies with two continuous variables usually named the x-values and y-values a linear relation between the two variables can be assessed with the help of the Pearson correlation coefficient R. R is a measure of strength of association and is often mathematically defined as:

$$\text{covariance}(x,y) / [\text{standard deviation } x . \text{standard deviation } y].$$

The best fit regression line provides for every x-value the best predictable y-value. The better the association the better one variable determines the other. R varies from −1 to +1.

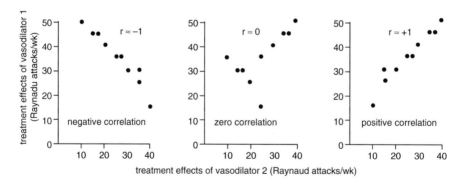

The above equation is used to assess whether the magnitude of R and its 95% confidence interval (the alternative hypothesis H1) is significantly different from zero and the same 95% confidence interval (the null hypothesis H0). Assuming normality, analysis of variance is used for computation. Instead of this also a Bayesian analysis of linear correlation is possible. It assesses the magnitude of the

© Springer International Publishing AG, part of Springer Nature 2018
T. J. Cleophas, A. H. Zwinderman, *Modern Bayesian Statistics in Clinical Research*,
https://doi.org/10.1007/978-3-319-92747-3_11

Bayes factor (BF). A BF smaller than "one" supports the above alternative hypothesis (H1), while a BF larger than "one" supports the above null hypothesis (H0). The BF is computed as the ratio of two likelihood distributions, that of the posterior and the prior likelihood distribution. The posterior is modeled from the computed Pearson correlation coefficient with its mode as maximum of the likelihood distribution. As prior a noninformative uniform prior can be applied. The computation of BF requires integrations for accuracy purposes. But, then, it can be used as a statistical index for quantifying the amount of support in favor H1 and H0. Advantages of the Bayesian approach may include.

1. A better underlying structure of the H1 and H0 may be provided.
2. Maximal likelihoods of likelihood distributions are not always identical to the mean effect of traditional tests, and this may be fine, because biological likelihoods may better fit biological questions than numerical means of non-representative subgroups do.

However, in spite of this, nobody knows for sure why likelihood distributions may better than normal distributions estimate uncertainties in statistical test results. So, why not use both of them for analyzing the same data example. The current chapter will show and compare the results of traditional Pearson correlation and Bayesian Pearson correlation analysis.

11.2   Introduction

The underneath table gives in 35 constipated patients the effect of numbers of monthly stools on a new laxative as assessed versus the effect of a standard laxative bisacodyl in a double blind crossover design. The patients that responded better on standard, also did so on the novel compound.

Patient no.	New laxative	Bisacodyl
1.	24,00	24,00
2.	30,00	13,00
3.	25,00	15,00
4.	35,00	10,00
5.	39,00	9,00
6.	30,00	10,00
7.	27,00	8,00
8.	14,00	5,00
9.	39,00	39,00
10.	42,00	42,00
11.	41,00	11,00
12.	38,00	11,00
13.	39,00	12,00
14.	37,00	10,00

15.	47,00	18,00
16.	30,00	30,00
17.	36,00	12,00
18	12,00	4,00
19.	26,00	10,00
20.	20,00	8,00
21.	43,00	16,00
22.	31,00	15,00
23.	40,00	14,00
24.	31,00	7,00
25.	36,00	12,00
26.	21,00	6,00
27.	44,00	19,00
28.	11,00	5,00
29.	27,00	8,00
30.	24,00	9,00
31.	40,00	15,00
32.	32,00	7,00
33.	10,00	6,00
34.	37,00	14,00
35.	19,00	7,00

new laxative = numbers of stools per month on the new laxative
bisacodyl = numbers of stools per month on the standard laxative bisacodyl

A traditional Pearson correlation analysis with the standard on the x-axis and the new laxative on the y-axis was performed. SPSS statistical software was applied. The data file entitled "chap11" is in extras.springer.com, and is first opened in your computer mounted with SPSS statistical software version 25 with the module Advanced Statistics included.

11.3   Traditional Analysis of Pearson Linear Correlation Analysis

Command:
click Analyze....Regression....Linear Regression....Dependent Variable: enter newlaxative data....Independent Variable (s): enter bisacodyl data....click OK.

The underneath tables are in the output.
Model summary

Model	R	R square	Adjusted R square	Std. error of the estimate
1	0.483[a]	0.233	0.210	8.86135

[a]Predictors: (constant), bisacodyl2

ANOVA[a]

Model		Sum of squares	df	Mean square	F	Sig.
1	Regression	788,894	1	788,894	10.047	0.003[b]
	Residual	2591,277	33	78,524		
	Total	3380,171	34			

[a]Dependent variable: newlaxative
[b]Predictors: (constant), bisacodyl2

Coefficients[a]

Model		Unstandardized coefficients		Standardized coefficients	t	Sig.
		B	Std. error	Beta		
1	(Constant)	23.487	2.743		8.561	0.000
	bisacodyl2	0.553	0.174	0.483	3.170	0.003

[a]Dependent variable: newlaxative

The correlation coefficient (R or r) between the bisacodyl and the new laxative effects is pretty large: $R = 0.483$, with an F-statistic of 10.047, significantly different from zero at a $p = 0.003$ level. A Bayesian analysis of the Pearson correlation will now be performed to find out whether the Bayes factor and posterior distribution are in agreement with the traditional Pearson correlation analysis. The null hypothesis of no difference from a correlation of zero between new and old treatment has already been assessed, and has already been rejected.

11.4   Bayesian Analysis of Pearson Linear Correlation

Command:
Analyze....Bayesian   Statistics....Test   Variable(s):   newlaxative, bisacodyl....Bayesian Aalysis: Use Both Methods....click Criteria: default settings....click Continue....click Priors: Uniform....click continue....click OK.

The underneath tables are in the output.

Bayes factor inference on pairwise correlations[a]

		newlaxative	bisacodyl2
newlaxative	Pearson correlation	1	0.483
	Bayes factor		0.105
	N	35	35
bisacodyl2	Pearson correlation	0.483	1
	Bayes factor	0.105	
	N	35	35

[a]Bayes factor: null versus alternative hypothesis

Posterior distribution characterization for pairwise correlations[a]

			newlaxative	bisacodyl2
newlaxative	Posterior	Mode		0.478
		Mean		0.446
		Variance		0.017
	95% Credible interval	Lower Bound		0.183
		Upper Bound		0.685
	N		35	35
blsacodyl2	Posterior	Mode	0.478	
		Mean	0.446	
		Variance	0.017	
	95% Credible interval	Lower Bound	0.183	
		Upper Bound	0.685	
	N		35	35

[a]The analyses assume reference priors (c = 0)

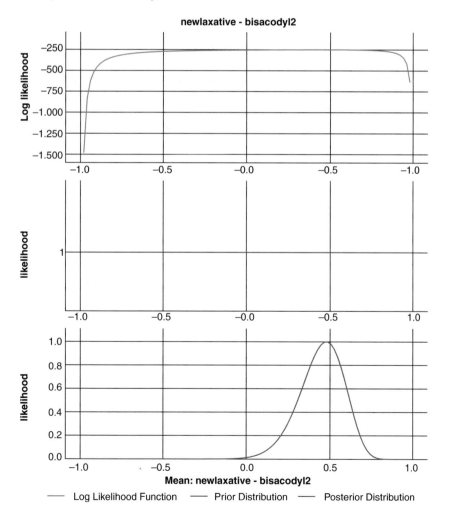

Bayes factor	Evidence category	Bayes factor	Evidence category	Bayes factor	Evidence category
>100	Extreme evidence for H0	1–3	Anecdotal evidence for H0	1/30 to 1/10	Strong evidence for H1
30–100	Very strong evidence for H0	1	No evidence	1/100 to 1/30	Very strong evidence for H1
10–30	Strong evidence for H0	1/3 to 1	Anecdotal evidence for H1	1/100	Extreme evidence for H1
3–10	Moderate evidence for H0	1/10 to 1/3	Moderate evidence for H1		

The Bayes factor was estimated as the ratio of likelihoods supporting the null versus the alternative hypothesis, or supporting no difference from an r-value of zero and the computed r-value of 0.483.

A Bayes factor of 0.105 means pretty strong support for the alternative hypothesis (an r-value significantly better than zero), and extreme lack of support for the null hypothesis (an r-value not different from zero). What does the Bayesian analysis tell which we did not yet know. We so far could reject the null hypothesis of no correlation at all. We could so far not state that H1 is true, because this was not assessed with traditional testing.

The posterior likelihood distribution was based on the measured parameters of interest after integrating out nuisance parameter. It was slightly skewed to the right with a mode of 0.478.

The maximum of the posterior likelihood distribution was 0.478 with 95% credible interval

$$0.183 \text{ to } 0.685.$$

This was less wide than the 95% confidence interval of the traditional Pearson linear correlation which was

$$0.483 \pm 2 \times \left[\left(4.83 \times 0.553 \right) / 0.174 \right] =$$
$$0.483 \pm 2 \times 0.1535 =$$
$$\text{between } 0.176 \text{ and } 0.790.$$

Thus, the Bayesian analysis provided slightly better statistics than did the traditional Pearson correlation analysis.

For Bayesian Pearson correlations reference priors may be adequately used. Reference priors belong to the class of noninformative priors that are inferred from beta or gamma distributions.

Reject H1

Bayes Factor	Evidence Category	Bayes Factor	Evidence Category	Bayes Factor	Evidence Category
>100	Extreme Evidence for H0	1-3	Anecdotal Evidence for H0	1/30-1/10	Strong Evidence for H1
30-100	Very Strong Evidence for H0	1	No Evidence	1/100-1/30	Very Strong Evidence for H1
10-30	Strong Evidence for H0	1/3-1	Anecdotal Evidence for H1	1/100	Extreme Evidence for H1
3-10	Moderate Evidence for H0	1/10-1/3	Moderate Evidence for H1		

Reject H0

With a BF of 0.105 rejection of the null hypothesis is supported, as shown above. This is a result similar to that of the traditional Pearson correlation assessment with an R value 0.483 and a p-value of 0.003.

11.5 Conclusion

This chapter assesses Bayesian Pearson correlations. They performed well and provided even slightly better sensitivity than traditional Pearson correlations did.

With modern Bayesian statistics likelihood distributions are the main probability distribution model. It is mostly based on the Cauchy distribution, a member of the family of the alpha distributions, and the distribution that best describes the ratio of two normal distributions or two likelihood distributions. Bayes factors have a Cauchy distribution, and cannot be numerically analyzed with standard Gaussian approximation methods. Fortunately, pretty good numerical results are obtained by integrations that integrate out nuisance variables like noninformative priors or lacking priors.

Advantages of the Bayesian approach may include.

1. A better underlying structure model of the H1 and H0 may be provided.
2. Bayesian tests work with 95% credible intervals that are usually somewhat wider and this may reduce the chance of statistical significances with little clinical relevance.

3. Maximal likelihoods of likelihood distributions are not always identical to the mean effect of traditional tests, and this may be fine, because biological likelihoods may better fit biological questions than numerical means of non-representative subgroups do.
4. Bayes uses ratios of likelihood distributions rather than ratios of Gaussian distributions, which are notorious for ill data fit.
5. Bayesian integral computations are very advanced, and, therefore, give optimal precisions of complex functions, and better so than traditional multiple mean calculations of non representative subsamples do.
6. With Bayesian testing type I and II errors need not being taken into account.

The Bayes factor (BF) in this chapter's example of 0.103 suggests that the Bayesian Pearson correlation analysis provides similar sensitivity of testing as that of the traditional Pearson correlation.

On a continuous line of Bayes factors from 1.0 to 0.0 our Bayes factor is in the right end.

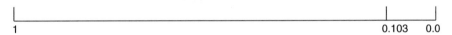

On a continuous line of p-values from 0.05 to 0.0 our p-value is similarly very much on the right end.

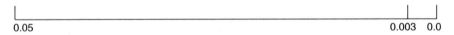

The BF of 0.103 is, equally, closer to right end side of 0.0, as the p-value of 0.003 is to right end side of 0.0. The BF and p-value provided approximately similarly sensitive statistics here.

Suggested Reading[1,2]

Statistics applied to clinical studies 5th edition, 2012
Machine learning in medicine a complete overview, 2015
SPSS for starters and 2nd levelers 2nd edition, 2015
Clinical data analysis on a pocket calculator 2nd edition, 2016
Understanding clinical data analysis from published research, 2016
Modern Meta-analysis, 2017
Regression Analysis in Clinical Research, 2018

---

[1] To readers requesting more background, theoretical and mathematical information of computations given, several textbooks complementary to the current production and written by the same authors are available.

[2] All of them have been written by the same authors, and they have been edited by Springer Heidelberg Germany.

Chapter 12
Bayesian Statistics: Markov Chain Monte Carlo Sampling

12.1 Background

Markov chain Monte Carlo (MCMC) procedures can be laid out as Bayesian tests. The Bayesian prior likelihood distribution of MCMC procedures could, for example, be a data file with missing data. The posterior likelihood distribution is based on the prior plus the MCMC computed imputation values.

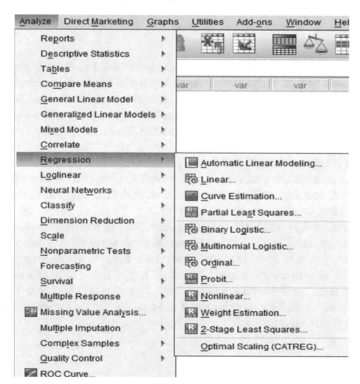

T. J. Cleophas, A. H. Zwinderman, *Modern Bayesian Statistics in Clinical Research*, https://doi.org/10.1007/978-3-319-92747-3_12

The above dialog box from SPSS statistical software is for producing Markov Chain Monte Carlo (MCMC) imputed data files, probably the best method for processing data files with missing data. Why so? With MCMC imputed data the imputated values are not used as constructed real values but rather as a device for representing missing data uncertainty.

MCMC modeling does not use maths for computing best fit values, but, rather, randomly sampled values from the data, the probabilities of which are iteratively tested against simulated values. This process stops, when the best fit probability has been obtained. MCMC modeling is like Monte Carlo (MC) modeling, but, while, with MC, simulations are independent, with MCMC, they are at desired levels of prior probabilities. In practice MCMC is more often successful in situations where MC does not work. The Markov Chain Monte Carlo (MCMC) procedure will be used in this chapter for the purpose of generating missing values for each variable in a data file by random sampling from the data. The MCMC procedure, thus, means that each sampled value is optimized by iteratively computing its probability against simulated random values, and after multiple iterations in this way the values with the best probabilities will be obtained. No further improvement is possible. In order to better explain the principles of the MCMC procedure, we need to describe the mechanisms of absorbing Markov chains.

12.2   Absorbing Markov Chains

Markov chains is a multiplicative predictive model where each subsequent probability is based on a prior data model. An example will be given. Patients with three states of treatment for a disease are checked after subsequent intervals. The data can be laid out in a data matrix, a so-called transition matrix. The states 1–3 may indicate the probability of treatment: 1 = no treatment, 2 = surgery, 3 = medicine. If you are in state 1 today, there will be a 0.3 = 30% probability that you will receive no treatment in the next interval, a 0.2 = 20% probability of surgery, and a 0.5 = 50% probability of medicine treatment. If you are still in state 1 (no treatment) after the first interval, then there will again be a 0.3 probability that this will be the same in the second etc. So, after 5 intervals the probability of being in state 1 equals $0.3 \times 0.3 \times 0.3 \times 0.3 \times 0.3 = 0.00243$. The probability that you will be in the states 2 or 3 is much larger, and there is something special about these states. Once you are in these states you will never leave them anymore, because the patients who were treated with either surgery or medicine are no longer followed in this study. That this happens can be observed from the matrix: if you are in state 2, you will have a probability of 1 = 100% to stay in state 2 and a probability of 0 = 0% not to do so. The same is true for the state 3.

State in current time	State in next period		
	1	2	3
1	0.3	0.2	0.5
2	0	1	0
3	0	0	1

Now we will compute what will happen with the probabilities of a patient in the state 1 after several intervals.

intervals = 4 month period	Probabilities of being in state:		
	state 1	state 2	state 3
1st	30%	20%	50%
2nd	$30 \times 0.3 = 9\%$	$20 + 0.3 \times 20 = 26\%$	$50 + 0.3 \times 50 = 65\%$
3rd	$9 \times 0.3 = 2.7\%$	$26 + 9 \times 0.2 = 27.8\%$	$65 + 9 \times 0.5 = 69.5\%$
4th	$3 \times 0.3 = 0.81\%$	$27.8 + 3 \times 0.2 = 28.4\%$	$69.5 + 3 \times 0.5 = 71.0\%$
5th	$0.9 \times 0.3 = 0.243\%$	$28.4 + 0.9 \times 0.2 = 28.6\%$	$71.0 + 0.9 \times 0.5 = 71.5\%$

Obviously, the probabilities of being in the states 2 or 3 will increase, though increasingly slowly, and the probability of being in state 1 is, ultimately, going to approximate zero. In clinical terms: postponing the treatment does not make sense, because everyone in the no treatment group will eventually receive a treatment and the ultimate probabilities of surgery and medicine treatment are approximately 29 and 71%. With larger matrices this method for calculating the ultimate chances is rather laborious. Matrix algebra offers a rapid method.

State in current time	State in next period				
	1	2 3			
1	[0.3]	[0.2 0.5]	matrix Q	matrix R
2	[0]	[1 0]	matrix O	matrix I
3	[0]	[0 1]		

The states are called transient, if they can change (the state 1), and absorbing if not (the states 2 and 3). The original matrix is partitioned into four submatrices, otherwise called the canonical form:

[0.3]	Upper left corner: This square matrix Q can be sometimes very large with rows and columns respectively presenting the transient states.
[0.2 0.5]	Upper right corner: This R matrix presents in rows the probability of being absorbed from the transient state.
[1 0] [0 1]	Lower right corner: This identity matrix I presents rows and columns with probabilities of being in the absorbing states, the I matrix must be adjusted to the size of the Q matrix (here it will look like [1] instead of [1 0]).
[0] [0]	Lower left corner. This is a matrix of zeros (0 matrix).

From the above matrices a fundamental matrix (F) is constructed.

$$\left[\left(\text{matrix I}\right)-\left(\text{matrix R}\right)\right]^{-1}=\left[0.7\right]^{-1}=10/7$$

With larger matrices a matrix calculator, like the Bluebit Online Matrix Calculator can be used to compute the matrix to the -1 power by clicking "Inverse". The fundamental matrix F equals 10/7. It can be interpreted as the average time, before someone goes into the absorbing state ($10/7 \times 4$ months $= 5.714$ months). The product of the fundamental matrix F and the R matrix gives more exact probabilities of a person in state 1 ending up in the states 2 and 3.

$$\text{F}\times\text{R}=\left(10/7\right)\times\left[0.2\ 0.5\right]=\left[2/7\ \ 5/7\right]=\left[0.285714\ \ \ 0.714286\right].$$

The two latter values add up to 1.00, which indicates a combined chance of ending up in an absorbing state equal to 100%.

12.3   Markov Chain Monte Carlo (MCMC) Sampling, Data Example

Instead of exact probabilities of some outcome in the next predictive interval, like the ones given in the above example, an outcome can be obtained differently. The MCMC procedure means that each sampled value is optimized by iteratively computing its probability against simulated random values, and after multiple iterations in this way the values with the best probabilities hopefully will be obtained. No further improvement is possible. An example will be given. Health related quality of life in small employers may be reduced. In a study of 500 small employers the effects on health related quality of life of various predictors including

1 age
2 chronic medications
3 income
4 people employed
5 chronic diseases

were assessed. The above variables were pretty significant. Also, many missing data were in the study, and a MCMC multiple imputations analysis was performed. We will use SPSS statistical software for data analysis. The data file entitled "chap12" is in extras.springer.com, and is opened in SPSS mounted with the multiple imputations submodule. Click Analyze, and the underneath dialog box comes up.

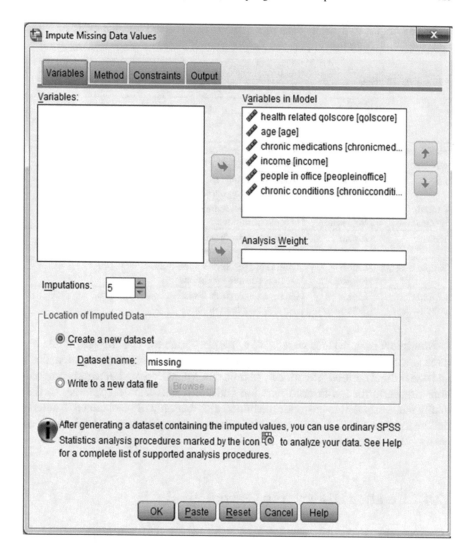

Command:

Analyze....click Multiple Imputations....click Impute Missing Data Values.... Variables: enter health related qolscore, age, chonic medications, income, people in office, chronic conditions....imputations: enter 5....mark Create a new data set....Dataset name: enter for example "missing"....click Method....mark Custom....mark Fully conditional specification MCMC....click Output....mark Create iteration history....Dataset name: enter for example "missing2"....click OK.

In the output two novel data files have been included entitled "missing" and "missing2". Also in the output was the underneath table.

Imputation models

	Model			
	Type	Effects	Missing values	Imputed values
Health related qolscore	Linear Regression	Age, chronic medications, income, people in office, chronic conditions	12	60
Age	Linear Regression	Qolscore, chronic medications, income, people in office, chronic conditions	11	55
Chronic medications	Linear Regression	Qolscore, age, income, people in office, chronic conditions	81	405
Income	Linear Regression	Qolscore, age, chronic medications, people in office, chronic conditions	91	455
People in office	Linear Regression	Qolscore, age, chronic medications, income, chronic conditions	49	245
Chronic conditions	Linear Regression	Qolscore, age, chronic medications, income, people in office	18	90

Multiple missing values were in all of the six variables. The "missing2" file has three new variables, two nominal entitled "imputations" and "summary statistics", and one ordinal entitled "iterations". In order for MCMC to work integral computations are performed with each iteration and the results should converge, so that finally the best possible posterior likelihood distribution will be obtained. An iteration history command is also available in the software program, and will be given next.

12.4   Iteration History with Ggraph

Ggraphs, otherwise called ggplots, are 2 dimensional plots of a graph with nodes and edges having x and y coordinates. Ggraphs is an abbreviation of "grammar of graphics for graphs and networks". In computer terminology ggraphs are API (application printing interface) tailored in order to draw complex networks of related nodes layer by layer. We will now use SPSS statistical software to help us draw a ggraph of five iteration histories of Monte Carlo generated missing values, using the above data example once more.

Command:
click Graph....Chart Builder....Gallery....click Line....select Multiple line....move to Chart....Y-Axis?: enter health related qolscore....X-Axis?: enter Iteration

Number....Set Color?: enter Imputation Number....Groups/Point ID: click....
mark Rows panel variable....Panel?: enter Summary Statistic....In Element
Properties: click OK.

In the output the underneath "ggraph" (or "ggplot"), with nodes and connections,
the iteration patterns of the means and standard deviations of the main outcome
variable are given. Particularly, the standard deviations tend to converge already
after ten iterations. Sometimes, more iterations may be needed in order for conver-
gence to take place.

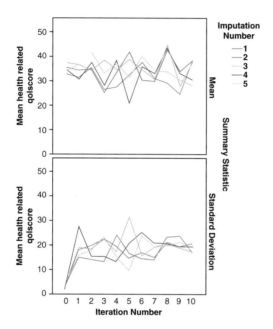

The "missing" dat)a file is also in our output. It looks much like the original data
file but has included a variable entitled "Imputation_number". Also it has a sample
size of 3000 instead of the 500 from the original data file. We will perform a regression analysis of this imputated data file. For that purpose common commands must
be given. However, the multiple imputations regression requires a different icon as
automatically shown in the Impute Missing Data Values dialog box (see
underneath).

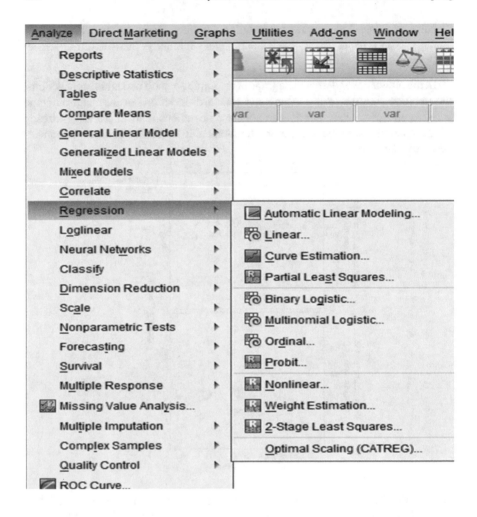

12.5   Bayesian Analysis of Imputated Models

The "missing" data file will now be applied for analyses of the five imputated models.

Traditional commands can be given. Our outcome variable "health related quality of life" is continuous. Therefore a linear regression can be performed.

Command
Analyze....Regression....click Linear (with novel icon as shown above)....
Dependent: enter health related qolscore....Independent (s): enter age, chronic medications, income, people in office, chronic conditions....Case Labels: Imputation Number....click OK.

The underneath tables are in the output.

Model summary[a]

Imputation number	Model	R	R square	Adjusted R square	Std. error of the estimate
Original data	1	,533[b]	,284	,271	17,678
1	1	,596[c]	,356	,349	16,935
2	1	,567[b]	,322	,315	17,436
3	1	,594[c]	,353	,346	16,995
4	1	,586[c]	,343	,337	17,013
5	1	,580[b]	,336	,329	17,199

[a]Dependent Variable: health related qolscore
[b]Predictors: (Constant), chronic conditions, income, chronic medications, age, people in office
[c]Predictors: (Constant), chronic conditions, income, chronic medications, people in office, age

ANOVA[a]

Imputation number	Model	Model	Sum of squares	df	Mean square	F	Sig.
Original data	1	Regression	34098,520	5	6819,704	21,823	,000[b]
		Residual	85937,274	275	312,499		
		Total	120035,794	280			
1	1	Regression	78237,807	5	15647,561	54,558	,000[c]
		Residual	141683,180	494	286,808		
		Total	219920,987	499			
2	1	Regression	71256,396	5	14251,279	46,876	,000[b]
		Residual	150185,509	494	304,019		
		Total	221441,905	499			
3	1	Regression	77856,574	5	15571,315	53,909	,000[c]
		Residual	142689,576	494	288,845		
		Total	220546,150	499			
4	1	Regression	74777,895	5	14955,579	51,669	,000[c]
		Residual	142987,414	494	289,448		
		Total	217765,310	499			
5	1	Regression	73964,153	5	14792,831	50,008	,000[b]
		Residual	146129,155	494	295,808		
		Total	220093,308	499			

[a]Dependent Variable: health related qolscore
[b]Predictors: (Constant), chronic conditions, income, chronic medications, age, people in office
[c]Predictors: (Constant), chronic conditions, income, chronic medications, people in office, age

Coefficients[a]

Imputation number	Model		Unstandardized coefficients		Standardized coefficients	t	Sig.
			B	Std. error	Beta		
Original data	1	(Constant)	22,184	5,411		4,100	,000
		Age	−,147	,146	−,080	−1,007	,315
		Chronic medications	,950	,157	,377	6,055	,000
		Income	−,014	,014	−,064	−1,007	,315
		People in office	,767	,172	,356	4,459	,000
		Chronic conditions	,215	,725	,016	,297	,767
1	1	(Constant)	18,520	3,655		5,067	,000
		Age	−,011	,098	−,007	−,110	,912
		Chronic medications	,708	,096	,348	7,388	,000
		Income	−,026	,011	−,105	−2,446	,015
		People in office	,824	,114	,406	7,229	,000
		Chronic conditions	,675	,536	,048	1,260	,208
2	1	(Constant)	15,882	3,754		4,231	,000
		Age	,082	,099	,049	,822	,411
		Chronic medications	,661	,101	,319	6,531	,000
		Income	−,012	,011	−,052	−1,093	,275
		People in office	,675	,123	,331	5,485	,000
		Chronic conditions	,722	,549	,051	1,314	,189
3	1	(Constant)	13,941	3,633		3,838	,000
		Age	,082	,096	,050	,855	,393
		Chronic medications	,738	,094	,365	7,822	,000
		Income	−,012	,011	−,048	−1,072	,284
		People in office	,638	,116	,315	5,481	,000
		Chronic conditions	1,224	,534	,086	2,293	,022
4	1	(Constant)	16,329	3,659		4,463	,000
		Age	,041	,097	,025	,419	,676
		Chronic medications	,747	,096	,372	7,783	,000
		Income	−,017	,011	−,067	−1,477	,140
		People in office	,682	,119	,334	5,752	,000
		Chronic conditions	,924	,535	,066	1,728	,085
5	1	(Constant)	14,059	3,668		3,832	,000
		Age	,117	,097	,071	1,204	,229
		Chronic medications	,675	,095	,327	7,074	,000
		Income	−,015	,011	−,061	−1,283	,200
		People in office	,677	,123	,333	5,489	,000
		Chronic conditions	,905	,547	,063	1,655	,099

[a]Dependent Variable: health related qolscore

The above tables show, that the r-square (squared correlation coefficients) values and the F-statistics of the imputated models are consistently better than those of the original regression model. SPSS provides adequate methods for pooling the results from the five imputation models, but this is not the objective of this chapter. More information on pooling methods for the purpose is available in SPSS' s Help directory, click "Analyzing Multiple Imputation Data". For the current chapter, rather than pooling, we will now use the imputation models for computing Bayes factors and assessing whether null and alternative hypotheses are, better than the original data, supported after data imputation.

With Bayesian statistics Bayes factors are used to assess whether H0 or H1 is better supported after data imputation or not. The Bayes factors of the data with missing data are calculated using the online Bayes Factor Calculators from Dept Psychol Sciences University Missouri, Columbia MO. Click Regression. Enter the requested data: sample sizes, covariates, squared correlation coefficients.

Rsquare =   0.284   for the original data

would mean that a

JZSBayes Factor equals **1.187963**; hardly in favor of H0.

In contrast.

Rsquare =   0.356   for the first imputation model

would mean that a

JZSBayes Factor equals **2.671638**; in favor of H0.

0.322   for the second imputation model

would mean that a

JZSBayes Factor equals **1.518048**; in favor of H0.

0.353   for the third imputation model

would mean that a

JZSBayes Factor equals **2.537739**; in favor of H0.

0.343   for the third imputation model

would mean that a

JZSBayes Factor equals **2.142738**; in favor of H0.

0.336   for the fifth imputation model

would mean that a

JZSBayes Factor equals **1.90718**; in favor of H0.

JZS = Jeffrey Zellner Siow Bayes factor. The Bayes factors (BFs) of the imputated models are, like the F-statistics of the traditional Anovas, generally, twice the size of those of the original data models. All of the five imputation models provided not only better traditional statistics, but also better JZS Bayes factors turning the likelihood distribution in favor of H1 (BF $\approx$ 1, no effect) into that of H0 (BF $\approx$ 2–3, real effect). Jeffreys Zellner Siow priors have also been used in the Chaps. 7 and 8.

12.6 Conclusion

Markov chain Monte Carlo (MCMC) procedures can be laid out as Bayesian tests. The Bayesian prior likelihood distribution of MCMC procedures could, for example, be a data file with missing data. The posterior likelihood distribution is based on the prior plus the MCMC computed imputation values. SPSS statistical software provides a special dialog box for the purpose. MCMC sampling involves multiplicative predictive models where each subsequent probability is based on a prior data model. An example was given. Patients with three states of treatment for a disease were checked after subsequent intervals. Instead of exact probabilities of some outcome in the next predictive interval, like the ones given in the above example, an outcome can obtained differently. With MCMC procedures randomly sampled values from your data are, prior to imputation in your data file, optimized by iteratively computing its probability against simulated random values, and after multiple iterations in this way the values with the best probabilities will be obtained. No further improvement is possible.

With Bayesian statistics Bayes factors are used to assess whether H0 or H1 is better supported after data imputation or not. The Bayes factors of the data samples with missing data were calculated using the online Bayes Factor Calculators from Dept Psychol Sciences University Missouri, Columbia MO. Click Regression. Enter the requested data: sample sizes, covariates, squared correlation coefficients. The Bayes factors (BFs) of the imputated models are, like the F-statistics of the traditional Anovas, over twice the size of those of the original data models. All of the five imputation models provided not only better traditional statistics, but also better JZS Bayes factors turning the likelihood distribution in favor of H1 (BF $\approx$ 1, no effect) into that of H0 (BF $\approx$ 2–3, real effect). Jeffreys and Jeffreys Zellner Siow priors have also been used in the Chaps. 7 and 8.

Suggested Reading[1,2]

Statistics applied to clinical studies 5th edition, 2012,
Machine learning in medicine a complete overview, 2015,
SPSS for starters and 2nd levelers 2nd edition, 2015,
Clinical data analysis on a pocket calculator 2nd edition, 2016,
Understanding clinical data analysis from published research, 2016,
Modern Meta-analysis, 2017,
Regression Analysis in Clinical Research, 2018.

---

[1] To readers requesting more background, theoretical and mathematical information of computations given, several textbooks complementary to the current production and written by the same authors are available.

[2] All of them have been written by the same authors, and they have been edited by Springer Heidelberg Germany.

Chapter 13
Bayes and Causal Relationships

13.1 Background

The current search for causal relationships with Bayesian structural equation modelings will be addressed in this chapter as an example where Bayesian methodologies successfully helped fostering the deepest enigma of mankind, the proof of causality. We do hope, that this chapter will be helpful to the medical and health community for which the dedication to the search for causalities is more vital than it is for most other disciplines. Regressions tell us something about relationships causal or not. For example, time- or place-related phenomena have a strong relationship, but are usually not causally related. A relationship does not cause causalities, although causality does cause relationships. The search for causal relationships is a never ending biased exercise of mankind, and regressions have often been erroneously interpreted. However, multistage regressions like the ones routinely used with path analysis and partial correlations may be a first step in the right direction.

13.2 Path Statistics

Path statistics uses add-up regression coefficients for better estimation of multiple step relationships. Because regression coefficients have the same unit as their variable, they can not be added up unless multiplied by the ratio of standard deviations. Standardized regression coefficients are, otherwise, called path statistics. The underneath figure gives a path diagram of data. We should add that standardized B-values (regression coefficients) are routinely provided in the output of any regression analysis given by statistical software programs. The relationship between standardized and unstandardized B-values is given underneath:

$$\text{Standardized B} = \text{unstandardized B} \times SD_x / SD_y.$$

© Springer International Publishing AG, part of Springer Nature 2018

T. J. Cleophas, A. H. Zwinderman, *Modern Bayesian Statistics in Clinical Research*,
https://doi.org/10.1007/978-3-319-92747-3_13

SD = standard deviation, B = regression coefficient. A convenient property of the standardized B is that it has a variance of 1, and that its unit is not grams, mmols, mms etc but rather SE (standard error) units. Standardized B-values can therefore be added, subtracted, multiplied etc.

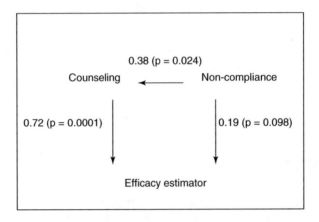

In the above table the standardized regression coefficients are added to the arrows. Single path analysis may give a standardized regression coefficient of 0.19. This underestimates the real effect of non-compliance on the efficacy estimator. Two step path analysis is more realistic and shows that the add-up path statistic is larger and equals

$$0.19 + 0.38 \times 0.72 = 0.46.$$

The two-path statistic of 0.46 is a lot better than the single path statistic of 0.19 with an increase of 60%.

It is easy to demonstrate that multiple steps provide a more sensitive prediction than a single step model does, particularly if they do statistically significantly so. And multiple paths similarly do so as compared to single paths. A series of significantly positive-related events interpreted as a possibly causal pathway, will be more easily believed, than the results of multiple independent predictors in a multiple regression analysis will be.

Multistep regressions are the basis of path analysis and path analysis is the basis of Bayesian networks using structural equation modeling (SEM). They will be visualized with DAGs, directed acyclic graphs, with arrows meant to indicate causality. If SEMs include

latent factors (unmeasured variables inferred from measured variables) as predictors, we will call it:

factor analysis if unsupervised (i.e., no dependent variable);
partial least squares if supervised;
discriminant analysis if like the above two but including a grouping variable.

manifest factors (variables), we will call it:

multistage regressions which might include flawed predictors, given pejorative names, like problematic predictors, multicollinear predictors, indirect predictors.

Bayesian networks do not necessarily use traditional Bayesian statistics, i.e., posterior and prior odds. Instead they use the methodologies of more modern Bayesian statistics, that is, conditional and marginal probability distributions (running from 0 to 1), and likelihood distributions (even running from 0 to ∞).

Finally, DAGs use arrows to indicate causal pathways, and these arrows are often called edges. The variables in the DAG are called nodes. DAGs are increasingly sophisticated. The term arrow is replaced with edge:

(1)   edges that are unidirectional,   have 1 vertex
(2)   "   undirectional,   have no vertex
(3)   "   bidirectional,   have 2 vertices
(4)   "   empty,   have neither edge nor vertex.

The above fourth type indicates no significant correlation between two variables. More information of how DAGs can be described in the form of conditional likelihoods are in the next chapter.

13.3   Path Analysis

The two underneath equalities look much like one another, and this is not only textually so but also conceptually. Var = variable.

prior likelihood distribution × Bayes factor = posterior likelihood distribution

   path statistic 1 × path statistic 2 = effect of Var 1 through Var 2 on Var 3.

The first one is the standard equation of Bayesian statistics, the second one is the standard equation of path analysis. An example of a data file analyzed with a more complex path analysis will be given. for convenience the data file is in extras. springer.com, and is entitled "chap13-1".

A 35 patient data file summarizes between-variable relationships. The first 10 patient data are underneath.

var 1 = stools per month
var 2 = qol (quality of life score)
var 3 = counselings per month
var 4 = compliance = non-compliances with drug treatment

Var 1	2	3	4
24,00	69,00	8,00	25,00
30,00	110,00	13,00	30,00
25,00	78,00	15,00	25,00
35,00	103,00	10,00	31,00
39,00	103,00	9,00	36,00
30,00	102,00	10,00	33,00
27,00	76,00	8,00	22,00
14,00	75,00	5,00	18,00
39,00	99,00	13,00	14,00
42,00	107,00	15,00	30,00

The linear correlation coefficients between all of the variables are computed. They are equal to the standardized regression coefficients and are also called path statistics. Their units are SEM (standard error of the mean) units, and they can, therefore, conveniently be added up or subtracted, unlike usual regression coefficients that have the same units as those of the variables they stem from like mmol/l, mg, sec etc.

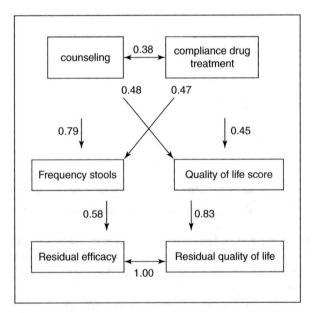

The above graph shows nine different path statistics computed as explained above.

A nice thing about path statistics is that they can be multiplied in order to compute indirect effects of one variable through another variable on a subsequent variable. For example:

effect of frequency of stools through counseling on quality of life score
$0.79 \times 0.48 = 0.38$
effect of frequency of stools through non-compliance on quality of life score
$0.45 \times 0.47 = 0.21$.

   As path statistics can be multiplied with one another, they can be used for assessing multiple step regressions and even as a nonmathematical method for performing complex multivariate regressions, the traditional mathematical alternative of which is much more complex.
   In this edition traditional and more modern versions of Bayesian statistics have been reviewed. It uses the equality "prior × Bayes-factor = posterior" where prior and posterior are short cuts for prior and posterior odds or likelihood distributions. Path statistics described as Bayesian statistics are underneath:

prior	× Bayes - factor	= posterior
path statistics 0.79	× 0.48	= 0.38
path statistics 0.45	× 0.47	= 0.21.

   Path statistics is the basis of structural equation modeling with directed acyclic graphs, and, given the similarity to Bayesian statistics, DAGs of structural equation models are currently commonly called Bayesian acyclic graphs and Bayesian network analysis.

13.4 Path Analysis and Partial Correlations

13.4.1 D-Separations

Causality in the above structural equation models is supported even more with the help of d-separations using partial correlation modeling. D-separations literally means separations based on dependencies. With d-separations the likelihood distribution of a predictor on an outcome is estimated on the condition that another predictor is held constant. Bayesian DAGs are here used as a way to figure out causal structures of biological models such that no experiments are needed. For example, the underneath DAG shows that blood sugar predicts stomach acidity, and stomach acidity predicts hunger.

$$\text{blood sugar} \rightarrow \text{stomach acidity} \rightarrow \text{hunger}$$

   The above simple DAG model asserts that blood sugar causes stomach acidity directly, and that stomach acidity causes hunger directly. This model implies that blood sugar and hunger are correlated. If acidity, being held constant, causes the significant correlation between blood sugar and hunger to disappear, then the

originally established correlation between blood sugar and hunger must have been
non-causal. Even with multiple predictors, partial correlations analysis is possible.
An example will be given.

Var 1 weightloss
Var 2 exercise
Var 3 calorieintake
Var 4 interaction
Var 5 age

1,00	0,00	1000,00	0,00	45,00
29,00	0,00	1000,00	0,00	53,00
2,00	0,00	3000,00	0,00	64,00
1,00	0,00	3000,00	0,00	64,00
28,00	6,00	3000,00	18000,00	34,00
27,00	6,00	3000,00	18000,00	25,00
30,00	6,00	3000,00	18000,00	34,00
27,00	6,00	1000,00	6000,00	45,00
29,00	0,00	2000,00	0,00	52,00
31,00	3,00	2000,00	6000,00	59,00
30,00	3,00	1000,00	3000,00	58,00
29,00	3,00	1000,00	3000,00	47,00
27,00	0,00	1000,00	0,00	45,00
28,00	0,00	1000,00	0,00	66,00
27,00	0,00	1000,00	0,00	67,00
28,00	0,00	1000,00	0,00	75,00
2,00	0,00	1000,00	0,00	64,00
30,00	0,00	1000,00	0,00	39,00
1,00	0,00	3000,00	0,00	65,00
3,00	0,00	3000,00	0,00	65,00
25,00	6,00	3000,00	18000,00	52,00
30,00	6,00	3000,00	18000,00	54,00
28,00	6,00	3000,00	18000,00	37,00
29,00	6,00	1000,00	6000,00	52,00
28,00	0,00	2000,00	0,00	65,00
29,00	3,00	2000,00	6000,00	49,00
30,00	3,00	1000,00	3000,00	50,00
30,00	3,00	1000,00	3000,00	51,00
27,00	0,00	1000,00	0,00	40,00
27,00	0,00	1000,00	0,00	46,00
26,00	0,00	1000,00	0,00	59,00
26,00	0,00	1000,00	0,00	53,00
1,00	0,00	1000,00	0,00	42,00
29,00	0,00	1000,00	0,00	53,00
2,00	0,00	3000,00	0,00	47,00
1,00	0,00	3000,00	0,00	54,00
28,00	6,00	3000,00	18000,00	35,00

27,00	6,00	3000,00	18000,00	46,00
30,00	6,00	3000,00	18000,00	56,00
27,00	6,00	1000,00	6000,00	39,00
29,00	0,00	2000,00	0,00	42,00
31,00	3,00	2000,00	6000,00	38,00
30,00	3,00	1000,00	3000,00	49,00
29,00	3,00	1000,00	3000,00	50,00
27,00	0,00	1000,00	0,00	51,00
28,00	0,00	1000,00	0,00	64,00
27,00	0,00	1000,00	0,00	65,00
28,00	0,00	1000,00	0,00	59,00
2,00	0,00	1000,00	0,00	53,00
30,00	0,00	1000,00	0,00	72,00
1,00	0,00	3000,00	0,00	65,00
3,00	0,00	3000,00	0,00	47,00
25,00	6,00	3000,00	18000,00	34,00
30,00	6,00	3000,00	18000,00	35,00
28,00	6,00	3000,00	18000,00	34,00
29,00	6,00	1000,00	6000,00	32,00
28,00	0,00	2000,00	0,00	62,00
29,00	3,00	2000,00	6000,00	53,00
30,00	3,00	1000,00	3000,00	47,00
30,00	3,00	1000,00	3000,00	54,00
27,00	0,00	1000,00	0,00	35,00
27,00	0,00	1000,00	0,00	46,00
26,00	0,00	1000,00	0,00	56,00
26,00	0,00	1000,00	45,00	23,00

The table gives the data of a simulated 64 patient study of the effects of exercise on weight loss with calorie intake as covariate. For convenience the data file is stored at extras.springer.com, and is entitled "chap13-2". We wish to perform a multiple linear regression of these data with weight loss as dependent (y) and exercise (x_1) and calorie intake (x_2) as independent predictor variables. Because the independent variables should not correlate too strong, first a correlation matrix is calculated as given below.

Correlations

		Weight loss	Exercise	Calorie intake
Weight loss	Pearson correlation	1	,405**	−,304*
	Sig. (2-tailed)		,001	,015
	N	64	64	64
Exercise	Pearson correlation	,405**	1	,390**
	Sig. (2-tailed)	,001		,001
	N	64	64	64

		Weight loss	Exercise	Calorie intake
Calorie intake	Pearson correlation	−,304[*]	,390[**]	1
	Sig. (2-tailed)	,015	,001	
	N	64	64	64

**Correlation is significant at the 0.01 level (2-tailed)
*Correlation is significant at the 0.05 level (2-tailed)

Correlation coefficients >0.80 or < −0.80 indicate collinearity, and that multiple regression is not valid. This is however, not so, and we can, thus, proceed.

Coefficients[a]

Model		Unstandardized coefficients		Standardized coefficients	t	Sig.
		B	Std. error	Beta		
1	(Constant)	34,279	2,651		12,930	,000
	Interaction	,001	,000	,868	3,183	,002
	Exercise	−,238	,966	−,058	−,246	,807
	Calorie intake	−,009	,002	−,813	−6,240	,000

[a]Dependent Variable: weight loss

The above table gives the results of the multiple linear regression. Both calorie intake and exercise are significant independent predictors of weight loss in the univariate models. However, exercise makes you hungry and patients on weight training may be inclined to reduce (or increase) their calorie intake. So, the presence of an interaction between calorie intake and exercise on weight loss is very well possible. In order to check this, an interaction variable (x_3 = calorie intake * exercise, with * symbol of multiplication) was added to the model. After the addition of the interaction variable to the regression model, exercise is no longer significant and interaction on the outcome is significant at p = 0.002. There is, obviously, interaction in the study, and the overall analysis of the data is no longer relevant. The best method to find the true effect of exercise the study should be repeated with calorie intake held constant. Instead of this laborious exercise, a partial correlation analysis with calorie intake held constant can be adequately performed, and would provide virtually the same result.

Model summary

Model	R	R square	Adjusted R square	Std. error of the estimate
1	,405[a]	,164	,151	9,73224

[a]Predictors: (Constant), exercise

Model summary

Model	R	R square	Adjusted R square	Std. error of the estimate
1	,644[a]	,415	,396	8,20777

[a]Predictors: (Constant), calorie intake, exercise

The above tables show that the simple linear regression between exercise and weight loss produced a correlation coefficient (r-value) of 0.405, and the multiple correlation coefficient, including calorie intake as additional predictor, was larger, 0.644. The r-square values are often interpreted as the % certainty about the outcome given by the regression analysis, and we can observe from the example that it rises from 0.164 to 0.415, meaning that with two predictors we have 42 instead of 16% certainty. The addition of the second independent variable provided 26% more certainty. But what about the correlation between the second variable (x_2) and the outcome (y). Is it equal to the square root of 0.26 = 0.51 (51%)? No, because multiple regression is a method that finds the best fit model for all of the data, and because, if you add new data, then all of the previously calculated relationships will change. The change in y caused by the addition of a second variable can be calculated by removing the amount of certainty provided by the presence of a novel variable.

$$\text{Novel y values} = \text{y values} - \text{mean } y - r_{yvsx2}\left(SD_y / SD_{x2}\right).$$

SD = standard deviation, vs = versus. Similarly the novel x_1 values can be calculated. Once this has been done for all individuals, an ordinary correlation between the novel values can be calculated. The novel correlation is interpreted as the correlation between y en x_1 with x_2 held constant, and is, otherwise, called the partial correlation.

With additional x variables, even higher-order partial correlations can be calculated, which are computationally very intensive, but calculations are pretty much the same. The interpretation is straightforward, the partial correlation between y en x_1 with two additional x variables is the correlation between y en x_1 with x_2 and x_3 held constant. What is the clinical relevance of partial correlations.

First, it can remove the effects of interactions of predictor variables on the outcome variable, and, thus, establish what would have happened, if there had been no interaction.

Second, it can be used to provide support for a causal relationship between variables: if with three paired variables one of three is held constant, and if this causes the previously significant correlation between the other two to disappear, then the originally established correlation between the latter two will probably be non-causal.

13.4.2 Partial Correlations Analysis

A partial correlation analysis will now be performed using SPSS, menu module Correlations. The data file called "chap13-2", available in extras.springer.com is opened it in your computer mounted with SPSS statistical software.

Command:
Analyze....Correlate....Partial....Variables: enter weight loss and exercise....
Controlling for: enter calorie intake....click OK.

Correlations

Control variables			Weight loss	Exercise
Calorie intake	Weight loss	Correlation	1,000	,596
		Significance (2-tailed)		,000
		df	0	61
	Exercise	Correlation	,596	1,000
		Significance (2-tailed)	,000	
		df	61	0

The above table shows that, with calorie intake held constant, exercise is a significant positive predictor of weight loss with a correlation coefficient of 0.596 and a p-value of 0.0001. It is interesting to observe that the partial correlation coefficient between weight loss and exercise is much larger than the simple correlation coefficient between weight loss and exercise (correlation coefficient = 0.405, former table). Why do we not have to account interaction with partial correlations. This is simply because, if you hold a predictor fixed, this fixed predictor can no longer change and interact in a multiple regression model.

13.4.3 Higher Order Partial Correlations Analysis

Instead of a single variable also multiple variables can be held constant in higher order partial correlation analyses. Age may affect all of the three variables already in the model. The effect of exercise on weight loss with calorie intake and age fixed is shown. The correlation coefficient is still very significant as shown in the underneath table.

Correlations

Control variables			Weight loss	Exercise
Age and calorie intake	Weight loss	Correlation	1,000	,541
		Significance (2-tailed)		,000
		df	0	60
	Exercise	Correlation	,541	1,000
		Significance (2-tailed)	,000	
		df	60	0

In the above partial correlations models the correlations between exercise and weight loss did not vanish. In contrast, the levels of correlation even increased as compared to the level of correlation in the univariate model of weight loss versus exercise. This would mean that the concept of causality is supported. A causal relationship between exercise and weight loss is supported.

13.5 Conclusion

The current search for causal relationships with Bayesian structural equation modelings is addressed in this chapter as an example where Bayesian statistics successfully helped fostering the deepest enigma of mankind, the proof of causality. Path analysis uses add-up sums and multiplications of standardized regression coefficients for better estimation of multiple step relationships. multiple steps provide a more sensitive prediction than a single step do, particularly if they do statistically significantly so. And multiple paths similarly do so, as compared to single paths. A series of significantly positive-related events interpreted as a possibly causal pathway, will be more easily believed, than the results of multiple independent predictors in a multiple regression analysis will be.

Bayes theorem although traditionally used for analyzing qualitative diagnostic tests is currently mostly applied for computation of Bayes factors. A Bayes factor is the ratio of two likelihood distributions, one of your data (posterior distribution), and one of relevant historical data (prior distribution).

The equality:

$$\text{"prior likelihood distribution} \times \text{Bayes factor = posterior likelihood distribution"}$$

looks much like the equalities used with path analysis, and this is not only textually so but also conceptually. An example with path statistics is underneath.

$$\text{"}\left[\text{path statistic 1}\right] \times \left[\text{path statistic 2}\right] = \left[\text{effect of Var 1 through Var 2 on Var 3}\right]\text{",}$$

where Var = variable.

In this chapter are examples of path analyses. With multiple variables they are called Bayesian networks, which are networks with a particular eye towards causality. Causality is even better substructured with partial correlation analysis of indirect predictors in a Bayesian network. The terms structural equation modeling and DAGs (directed acyclic graphs) are commonly applied within this context.

Suggested Reading[1,2]

Statistics applied to clinical studies 5th edition, 2012,
Machine learning in medicine a complete overview, 2015,
SPSS for starters and 2nd levelers 2nd edition, 2015,
Clinical data analysis on a pocket calculator 2nd edition, 2016,
Understanding clinical data analysis from published research, 2016,
Modern Meta-analysis, 2017,
Regression Analysis in Clinical Research, 2018.

---

[1]To readers requesting more background, theoretical and mathematical information of computations given, several textbooks complementary to the current production and written by the same authors are available.

[2]All of them have been written by the same authors, and they have been edited by Springer Heidelberg Germany.

Chapter 14
Bayesian Network

14.1 Introduction

A Bayesian network (BN) is a tool to describe and analyze multivariate distributions. The tool is member of the family of probabilistic graphical models. Despite its association, Bayesian networks do not necessarily use Bayesian statistical methods for data-analysis, the name refers rather to the way conditional and marginal probability distributions are related to each other. Bayesian networks are sometimes used in conjunction with Bayesian statistical methods, especially when prior knowledge is analyzed together with data, but this is not unique for BNs. Graphical models in general, and Bayesian networks too, have been proposed especially to deal with complex data (-analysis), and with an eye towards causal interpretations. This is achieved by combining graph theory, probability theory, statistics and computer science. Bayesian networks have been used in many different fields, for instance, in the Microsoft Windows system and the NASA mission control. In biomedicine the main applications seems to be in expert systems, in bioinformatics applications in genetics, and in identifying gene-regulatory networks.

14.2 Bayesian Networks for Cause Effect Modeling in Surveys

14.2.1 Example

In 600 patients, 70 years of age, a score sampling of factors predicting longevity was performed. The outcome was death after 10 years of follow-up. The first 12 patients are underneath, the entire data file is entitled "chap14-1", and is available at extras.springer.com. We will first perform a logistic regression of these data using SPSS statistical software. Start by opening SPSS. Enter the above data file.

© Springer International Publishing AG, part of Springer Nature 2018
T. J. Cleophas, A. H. Zwinderman, *Modern Bayesian Statistics in Clinical Research*,
https://doi.org/10.1007/978-3-319-92747-3_14

Variables					
1	2	3	4	5	6
death	econ	psychol	physic	family	educ
0	70	117	76	77	120
0	70	68	76	56	114
0	70	74	71	57	109
0	90	114	82	79	125
0	90	117	100	68	123
0	70	74	100	57	121
1	70	77	103	62	145
0	70	62	71	56	100
0	90	86	88	65	114
0	90	77	88	61	111
0	110	56	65	59	130
0	70	68	50	60	118

death (0 = no)
econ = economy score
psychol = psychological score
physic = physical score
family = familial risk score of longevity
educ = educational score

14.2.2 Binary Logistic Regression in SPSS

Command:
Analyze....Regression....Binary   Logistic....Dependent: enter   "death"....
Covariates: enter "econ, psychol, physical, family, educ"....OK.

The underneath output table shows the results. With $p < 0.10$ as cut-off for statistical significance, all of the covariates, except economical score, were significant predictors of longevity (death), although both negative and positive b-values were observed.

Variables in the equation

		B	S.E.	Wald	df	Sig.	Exp(B)
Step 1[a]	ecom	,003	,006	,306	1	,580	1,003
	psychol	−,056	,009	43,047	1	,000	,946
	physical	−,019	,007	8,589	1	,003	,981
	family	,045	,017	7,297	1	,007	1,046
	educ	,017	,009	3,593	1	,058	1,018
	Constant	−,563	,922	,373	1	,541	,569

[a]Variable(s) entered on step 1: ecom, psychol, physical, family, educ.

For these data we hypothesized that all of these scores would independently affect longevity. However, indirect effects were not taken into account, like the effect of psychological on physical scores, and the effect of family on educational scores etc. In order to assess both direct and indirect effects, a Bayesian network DAG (directed acyclic graph) was fitted to the data. The Konstanz Information Miner (Knime) was used for the analysis. In order to enter the SPSS data file in Knime, an excel version of the data file is required. For that purpose open the file in SPSS and follow the commands.

Command in SPSS:
click File....click Save as....in "Save as" type: enter Comma Delimited (*.csv).... click Save.

For convenience the excel file has been added to extras.springer.com, and is, just like the SPSS file, entitled "chap14-2".

14.2.3 Konstanz Information Miner (Knime)

In Google enter the term "knime". Click Download and follow instructions. After completing the pretty easy download procedure, open the knime workbench by clicking the knime welcome screen. The center of the screen displays the workflow editor like the canvas in SPSS Modeler it is empty., and can be used to build a stream of nodes, called workflow in knime. The node repository is in the left lower angle of the screen, and the nodes can be dragged to the workflow editor simply by left-clicking. The nodes are computer tools for data analysis like visualization and statistical processesKnime (Konstanz Information Miner). Node description is in the right upper angle of the screen. Before the nodes can be used, they have to be connected with the file reader and with one another by arrows drawn again simply by left clicking the small triangles attached to the nodes. Right clicking on the file reader enables to configure from your computer a requested data file....click Browse....and download from the appropriate folder a csv type Excel file. You are almost set for analysis now, but in order to perform a Bayesian analysis Weka software 3.6 for windows (statistical software from the University of Waikato (New Zealand) is requiredKnime (Konstanz Information Miner). Simply type the term Weka software, and find the site. The software can be freely downloaded from the internet, following a few simple instructions, and it can, subsequently, be readily opened in Knime. Once it has been opened, it is stored in your Knime node repository, and you will be able to routinely use it.

14.2.4 Knime Workflow

A knime workflow for the analysis of the above data example is built, and the final result is shown in the underneath figure

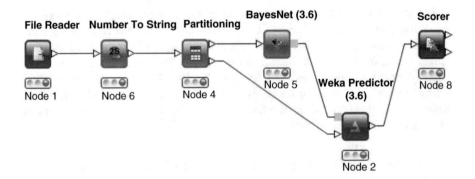

In the node repository click and type File Reader and drag to workflow editor in the node repository click again File reader....click the ESC button of your computer....in the node repository click again and type Number to String....the node is displayed....drag it to the workflow editor....perform the same kind of actions for all of the nodes as shown in the above figure....connect, by left clicking, all of the nodes with arrows as indicated above....click File Reader....click Browse....and type the requested data file ("longevity.csv")....click OK....the data file is given....right click all of the nodes and then right click Configurate and execute all of the nodes by right clicking the nodes and then the texts "Configurate" and "Execute"....the red lights will successively turn orange and then green....right click the Weka Predictor node.... right click the Weka Node View....right click Graph.

The underneath graph shows the Bayesian network obtained from the analysis.

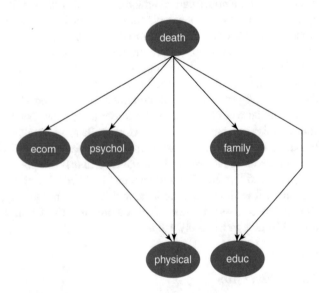

The best fitting DAG was, obviously, more complex than expected from the logistic model. Longevity was directly determined by all of the 5 predictors, but additional indirect effects were between physical and psychological scores, and between educational and family scores. In order to assess the validity of the Bayesian model, a confusion matrix and accuracy statistics were computed.

Right click the Scorer node....right click Confusion matrix

Confusion Matrix

Table "spec_name" - Rows: 2	Spec - Columns: 2	Properties	Flow Variables

Row ID	0	1
0	295	70
1	91	44

The observed and predicted values are summarized. Subsequently, right click Accuracy statistics.

Accuracy Statistics

Row ID	TruePo...	FalsePo...	TrueNe...	FalseN...	Recall	Precision	Sensitivity	Specifity
0	295	91	44	70	0.808	0.764	0.808	0.326
1	44	70	295	91	0.326	0.386	0.326	0.808
Overall	?	?	?	?	?	?	?	?

The sensitivity of the Bayesian model to predict longevity was pretty good, 80.8%. However, the specificity was pretty bad. "No deaths" were rightly predicted in 80.8% of the patients, "deaths", however, were rightly predicted in only 32.6% of the patients.

14.2.5   Discussion

Bayesian networks are probabilistic graphical models for assessing cause effect relationships. This example assesses if Bayesian networks was able to determine direct and indirect predictors of binary outcomes like morbidity/mortality outcomes. A longevity study was used for the purpose. Longevity is multifactorial, and logistic regression is adequate to assess the chance of longevity in patients with various predictor scores like physical, psychological, and family scores. However, factors may have both direct and indirect effects. A best fit Bayesian network demonstrated not only direct but also indirect effects of the factors on the outcome.

14.3   Bayesian Networks for Cause Effect Modeling in Clinical Trials

14.3.1   Example

The data that we will use here, comes from a randomized clinical trial that evaluated efficacy of pravastatin to reduce cardiovascular events, and to reduce the decrease of the diameter of coronary vessels (Jukema, Circulation 91:2528–2540). The trial consisted of a random sample of 884 men with cardiovascular heart disease and normal to moderately enhanced LDL-cholesterol levels. Patients were randomized between 20 mg pravastatin daily or placebo for 2 years. Outcome variables were the change in mean diameter of the coronary segments measured at baseline and after 2 years with coronary angiography, and occurrence of coronary events during follow-up (death, myocardial infarction, stroke, coronary intervention). Four hundred fifty patients were randomized to pravastatin treatment and 434 to placebo. At baseline there were no significant or substantial differences between the two groups with respect to age, baseline LDL- and HDL-cholesterol, smoking history, and current hypertension. Also the average diameter of the coronary vessels did not differ between the groups at baseline. After 2 years of follow-up the number of patients with a coronary event was significantly lower in the patients who were treated with pravastatin, the decrease of the diameter of the coronary vessels was also significantly lower, and the change of LDL- and HDL-cholesterol levels was also significantly larger in the statin treated patients. Statins were supposed to work mainly through improving lipid levels, which would, in turn, decrease the atherosclerotic process of lipid deposition in the wall of the coronary vessels. This process would, then, lead to lower risk of coronary events. This description forms a typical causal hypothesis that can be analyzed with graphical models. Underneath a patient characteristic table including the effect of treatment on risk of coronary event is given.

	Placebo(n = 434)	Pravast (n = 450)	P-value
Coronary Event: n (%)	79 (18%)	48 (11%)	0.001
Decrease of the mean: diameter of the coronary vessels (mm): mean (SD)	0.10 (0.21)	0.06 (0.19)	0.014
LDL-cholesterol decrease (mmol/L): mean (SD)	−0.04 (0.59)	1.23 (0.68)	<0.001
HDL cholesterol increase (mmol/L): mean (SD)	0.03 (0.13)	0.10 (0.16)	<0.001
Age (years): mean (SD)	56 (8)	57 (8)	0.26

	Placebo(n = 434)	Pravast (n = 450)	P-value
LDL-cholesterol level at baseline (mmol/L): mean (SD)	4.31 (0.78)	4.30 (0.78)	0.75
HDL-cholesterol level at baseline(mmol/L): mean (SD)	0.93 (0.23)	0.93 (0.23)	0.72
baseline mean diameter coronary vessels (mm): mean (SD)	2.82 (0.48)	2.80 (0.46)	0.46
Smoking ever: n (%)	376 (87%)	402 (89%)	0.22
Current hypertension: n (%)	134 (31%)	112 (25%)	0.06

14.3.2 Methodological Background of Bayesian Networks

Nodes and Edges

Bayesian networks are probabilistic graphical models and use graphical structures to represent knowledge. In particular _nodes_ and _edges_ are used, where a node represents a random variable and an edge between two nodes represents a probabilistic dependency between two variables. If edges are undirected the graphical models are usually called Markov networks of Markov random fields, but in Bayesian networks edges, usually, have direction and the graph is, then, called a directed acyclic graph (DAG). The multivariate distribution of the variables in the DAG can be represented efficiently, and the DAG provides also an easy way to estimate the data distributions.

Parent and Child Nodes

The directed edge from variable X_i to variable X_j represents the statistical dependence of X_j and X_i, but slightly stronger. The X_i is also defined to influence X_j or be X_j's parent (X_j is defined to be X_i's child). Or, in more general terms, X_j is X_i's descendant and X_i is X_j's ancestor. The DAG is acyclic, and that guarantees that a variable cannot be its own descendant or ancestor. A directed edge from X_i to X_j is often understood to represent a _causal_ relationship between the two variables X_i and X_j.

Path Analysis

For our data example, we can consider the graph in underneath figure. Three variables are connected with two arrows, that can be considered as path statistics
which are usually simple standardized linear regression coefficients. The Bayesian equality

$$prior \times Bayes factor = posterior$$

looks like

path statistic 1×path statistic 2 = effect of Var 1 through Var 2 on Var 3.

And this is not only textually, but also conceptionally so (Var = variable).

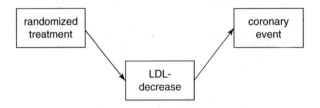

Directed Acyclic Graph

Instead of a path analysis the above graph is also called a simple directed acyclic graph (DAG). The simple DAG is of the causal effect of the statin treatment variable on LDL (low density lipoprotein) decrease and the occurrence of coronary events during the follow up of the clinical trial of patients with coronary heart disease. The directed edge between "randomized treatment" and "LDL-decrease" points to our expectation that the choice of treatment will influence how much LDL-cholesterol will decrease. The directed edge between "LDL decrease" and "coronary event" points to our expectation that the amount of LDL-decrease, in turn, will determine the risk of a coronary event. Thus, "randomized treatment" is an ancestor of both "LDL-decrease", and "coronary event", and "LDL-decrease" is also an ancestor of "coronary event".

Conditional Independence

BNs have rather simple conditional dependence and independence statements. The (directed) edge between "randomized treatment" and "LDL-decrease" signifies a direct dependence, namely that the distribution of the latter depends on the specific value of the former. But far more general, one may say that each variable is independent of its nondescendents in the graph *given* the state of its parents. Thus, "coronary event" is independent of "randomized treatment" *given* that the amount of "LDL-decrease" is known. Note that this particular DAG corresponds to the <u>causal</u> hypothesis that statin-treatment works only through lowering LDL-cholesterol level, and, thus, excludes a pleiotropic effect of statins.

Conditional Probabilities

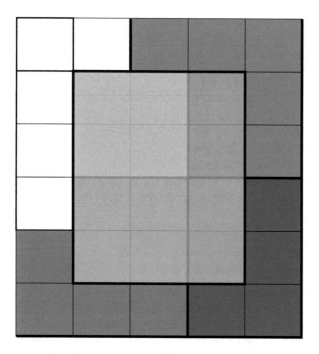

Conditional probabilities can be explained using partially overlapping colored squares like those given in the above graph. The blue and red areas are conditionally independent of the yellow area (Pr = probability, ∩ = together with, I = given). Area of overlap are 6 squares colored purple. Of the 12 squares colored yellow two of them have overlap with both the blue and the red area. This means.

$$\Pr\left(\text{red} \cap \text{blue} \,|\, \text{yellow}\right) = 2/12 \left(= 1/6\right).$$

Of the 12 yellow squares 4 are also red. This means:

$$\Pr\left(\text{red} \,|\, \text{yellow}\right) = 4/12 \left(1/3\right).$$

Of the 12 yellow squares 6 are also blue. This means:

$$\Pr\left(\text{blue} \,|\, \text{yellow}\right) = 6/12 \left(1/2\right).$$

Conditional Likelihoods

Conditional likelihoods are very much the same as conditional probabilities, but be careful. Likelihood may be synonymous to probabilities, but with statistical computations often standardized likelihoods are applied as obtained by dividing the observed likelihoods by the maximal likelihood of a likelihood distribution. Likelihoods of a likelihood distribution add up to 1, standardized likelihoods add up to >1 (see Chap. 1). With modern Bayesian statistics the latter are routinely used for computing the areas under the curves of the posterior and prior likelihood distributions (L = likelihood).

A Bayesian network is, in addition to a DAG, represented by a set of conditional standardized likelihood distributions that together describe the multivariate distribution $L(X,Y,Z)$ where X = "randomized treatment", Y = "LDL-decrease" and Z = "coronary event". The term standardized is often omitted. For the above DAG we can describe

$L(X,Y,Z)$ as the product
$L(X)*L(Y|X)*L(Z|Y)$, where
$L(Y|X)$ means the likelihood of Y given X.

Given that the randomized treatment is determined by chance, $L(X)$ would typically be described by a Bernoulli distribution with probability 0.5 (i.e. "throwing a coin"). LDL-decrease is a normal distributed quantity and $L(Y|X)$ would therefore be a conditional distribution usually described with ordinary linear regression, and, because coronary event is a binary variable, $L(Z|Y)$ would typically be described by logistic regression. Leaving out the directed edge from "randomized treatment" to "coronary event" means that $L(X,Y,Z)$ is less complex than a saturated model is. It means that one parameter less needs to be estimated from the data. BNs of many variables can benefit greatly from assuming clinically sound structures that are inferentially much easier, and results can be far more robust with far less variance. The complexity of the multivariate distribution modeled with a BN is quantified by the so-called *d-separation* statistic (see Chap. 13, section Bayes and Partial Correlations).

Marginalizations

Inference in a Bayesian network is done by marginalization, meaning that irrelevant variables are integrated or summed out. If the risk of a coronary event must be calculated for patients treated with pravastatin, this is calculated by

$L(Z|X=statin)$ =
$\int L(Z|Y=y)\, L(Y=y|X=statin)\, dy.$

Basically, the likelihood of a coronary event for all possible LDL-decreases $Y = y$ are considered (i.e. $L(Z|Y = y)$) and these likelihoods are averaged but weighted with the likelihood that such a LDL-decrease $Y = y$ is observed under statin treatment (i.e., $L(Y = y|X = statin)$). For a particular variable in a general Bayesian network this marginalization can be done through either its parents or its children, and the former is called *predictive support* or *top-down reasoning* while the latter is called *diagnostic support* or *bottom-up reasoning* (see next section).

Markov Chain Monte Carlo Sampling

Which strategy is chosen, is determined for opportunistic reasons, but if the Bayesian network is large, exact inference may be very hard involving multiple integrals or summations. Popular exact algorithms are message-passing, cycle-cutset and variable-elimination. Approximate algorithms are useful for large Bayesian networks and are mostly based on Monte Carlo sampling such as the Markov Chain Monte Carlo (MCMC) methods (see also the Chap. 12)

Bayesian Information Criterion

Learning a new BN from data presents several difficulties: the Bayesian network structure may be known or unknown, the shapes of the conditional distributions $L(X_j|X_i)$ and their parameters may be known or unknown, and the variables in the Bayesian network may be observed or only partially observed. Given a particular Bayesian network structure and appropriate data, the best parameters describing the multivariate distribution are found by maximization of the log-likelihood of the data. This is fully comparable to estimating any statistical model. For the Bayesian network in the above graph this would entail estimating the parameters of the linear regression model of LDL-decrease on randomized treatment and of the logistic regression model of coronary event on LDL-decrease. If the Bayesian network contains nodes for which no data is available, then the unobserved nodes must be partialed out. This can be done using MCMC methods or with expectation-maximization algorithms in less complex cases.

If the Bayesian network structure is unknown, the problem is, unfortunately, much harder, because the number of different DAGs with N variables is superexponential in N. In practice one then, usually, starts with a reasonably simple DAG (a naive Bayesian network for instance), and, then, adds those edges to the DAG that minimize some goodness of fit criterion such as the Akaike's or Bayesian Information Criterion (AIC/BIC). The AIC is computed from the equation

$$AIC = 2(\text{number of regressors} - \text{loglikelihood ratio}).$$

The loglikelihood ratio is the log transformed ratio of the observed likelihood and the maximal likelihood estimate (MLE) of the best fit statistical model chosen. The AIC can be used to estimate the goodness of fit of that model to your data. The smaller the AIC the better the fit. The AIC method is the approach we used for our example data.

Matlab Syntax Used

When using Matlab Bayes Net toolbox [code.google.com/p/bnt/], the following syntax commands from Matlab prompt should be given.

1. For model selection:

   P(DIG) = \int_{\theta}p(DIG),\theta)

2. For finding the best model:

   \sum_{k = 0}^n\choice{n}{k} = 2^n

3. For computing BIC values:

   \log\Pr(DIG)\approx\log\Pr(DIG).\hat{\Theta}_G) − \frac{\log N}{2} / #G

14.3.3   Results of Fitting a Bayesian Network to Our Example

For our data we hypothesized that the randomized treatment, pravastatin versus placebo, only affected the risk of coronary events through lowering LDL-cholesterol. We assumed that this, on its turn, would reduce the decrease of the diameters of the coronary vessels. We hypothesized, in addition, that smoking affected the diameters of the coronary vessels, and that hypertension had a direct effect on the risk of coronary events. The DAG is illustrated in the underneath graph.

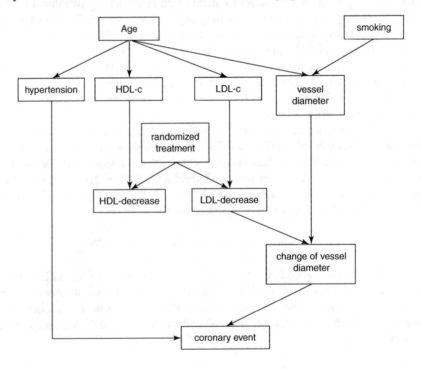

The above DAG corresponds with a Bayesian network in which the effect of statin treatment has a direct effect on LDL-cholesterol and no direct effect on the diameter of the coronary vessels nor direct effect on coronary events. The DAG has three parents, namely "age", "smoking", and "randomized treatment". The structure hypothesizes, that the difference between the risk of coronary event with placebo and with pravastatin ($p < 0.0001$, see table on the above third page of this chapter) will probably vanish by conditioning on the change of the vessel diameter. Similarly, the associations between age and smoking and coronary events will probably vanish after conditioning on hypertension and change of vessel diameter. The AIC values of the hypothesized DAG in the graph and of five different Bayesian networks are reported in the table below.

Nr	Model	AIC
0	As illustrated in Figure 16.2	13147.26
1	Model 0 plus direct effects of LDL- and HDL-cholesterol decreases on events	13145.15
2	Model 1 plus direct effect of randomized treatment on events	13139.49
3	Model 1 plus direct effect of randomized treatment on change of diameter	13143.06
4	Model 2 plus direct effect of randomized treatment on change of diameter	13135.29
5	Model 3 plus direct effects of smoking on events and change of diameter	13136.83

The optimal AIC value was, obviously, found for AIC number 4. In this model the conditional distribution of vessel-diameter-change depended directly on smoking and randomized treatment, and the risk of a coronary event depended on the amount of LDL- and HDL-cholesterol change, and, in addition, on the randomized treatment. This latter results may be interpreted as pleiotropic effects of pravastatin.

The best fitting DAG, the above number 4, was, thus, much more complicated than expected, involving dependencies between age and smoking, between smoking and baseline hypertension, LDL- and HDL-cholesterol, and of all of these on LDL- and HDL-cholesterol change and change of vessel diameter. Coronary event appeared, in contrast, to be dependent only on randomized treatment and not on LDL- or HDL-decrease.

14.3.4   Discussion

Bayesian Networks have obtained much enthusiasm in many applied research fields. The graphical interface has proved to be very helpful both in summarizing relationships between a large set of variables and for hypothesizing about causality. The graphical display has been adopted very widely, for instance, by biomolecular scientists to describe pathogenic and metabolic pathways. But the graphical tools have proved to be appealing in every applied field. The causal interpretation of BNs is (in contrast) somewhat problematic in biomedicine. Causality is difficult in biomedical research, because, often, confounding effects can not be ruled out in observational data, and it is very difficult to specify the influence of selection processes for any given sample of patients. It is also difficult to do controlled experiments with human subjects.

Apart from interpretations, BNs are very efficient to describe multivariate distributions. The structure makes inference of BNs often robust and it also reduces variance of estimated parameters. Thus BNs are often robust against overfitting. In case a new network is learned from a dataset, it is nevertheless highly recommended to perform some form of cross validation to assess reliability of the network.

Software for Bayesian networks are available in many computer programs. Several packages are available in the freeware/shareware R system [www.r-project.org, package: deal], several algorithms are offered in the weka package [weka.sourceforce.net] and the Matlab Bayes Net toolbox [code.google.com/p/bnt/].

In summary.

1. The graphical display of Bayesian networks has been adopted very widely, for instance, by biomolecular scientists to describe pathogenic and metabolic pathways.
2. The graphical tools have proved to be appealing in every applied field. The causal interpretation of BNs is (in contrast) somewhat problematic in biomedicine.
3. Causality is difficult in biomedical research, because, often, confounding effects can not be ruled out in observational data, and it is also difficult to do controlled experiments with human subjects.
4. Bayesian networks are very efficient to describe multivariate distributions. The structure makes inferences from Bayesian networks robust, reduces variances of estimated parameters, and is also robust against overfitting.

14.4   Bayesian Networks for Analyzing Meta-Data

14.4.1   Meta-Data from Lazarou-1

In a meta-analysis of Lazarou et al. studies were assessed for hospital admissions due to severe adverse effects (JAMA 1998; 279: 1200–5)

VAR 1	2	3	4
year of study	investigator type	study size	% admissions due to adverse effects
1995,00	2,00	379,00	5,30
1995,00	2,00	4031,00	4,40
1994,00	1,00	1024,00	10,30

VAR 1	2	3	4
year of study	investigator type	study size	% admissions due to adverse effects
1993,00	2,00	420,00	3,60
1981,00	1,00	815,00	14,80
1979,00	2,00	1669,00	16,80
1977,00	2,00	152,00	7,20
1977,00	1,00	334,00	10,20
1973,00	1,00	11526,00	22,50
1973,00	2,00	658,00	12,20
1971,00	2,00	8291,00	1,20
1970,00	1,00	939,00	10,50
1968,00	1,00	830,00	24,10
1967,00	1,00	267,00	10,90
1966,00	1,00	714,00	13,60
1966,00	1,00	900,00	10,80
1965,00	1,00	500,00	8,20
1964,00	1,00	1014,00	10,20

VAR = variable
%ADEs = percentage adverse drug effects
By clinicians = study performed by clinician investigators
Elderly = study of elderly patients

In the above 18 studies published 1964–1995, the percentage of hospital admission due severe adverse drug effects were assessed. The percentage of adverse drug admissions out of all of the admission was the main outcome measure. As this meta-analysis was very heterogeneous, a multiple linear regression was performed to find out what predictors may have influenced the outcome.

Coefficients[a]

Model		Unstandardized coefficients		Standardized coefficients	t	Sig.
		B	Std. error	Beta		
1	(Constant)	155,540	280,645		,554	,588
	Year of study	−,070	,143	−,128	−,487	,634
	Department	−5,418	3,148	−,453	−1,721	,107
	Study size	,000	,000	,172	,765	,457

[a]Dependent Variable: % severe

This multiple linear regression with percentage severe adverse events as outcome and three predictors, (1) year of study, (2) department (internal medicine or otherwise, and (3) study size, shows, that, with p = 0.15 as cut-off for statistical significance only the department (= type of investigator, internist or otherwise) is a significant predictor of percentage of adverse effects.

Next, we will perform a Bayesian network assessment, bottom-up reasoning, and we will use for the purpose the Knime and Weka software programs. In order for readers to perform their own analyses examples of step by step analyses are given in Machine learning in medicine a complete overview, the Chaps. 7, 70, 71, 74, Springer Heidelberg Germany, 2015, from the same authors.

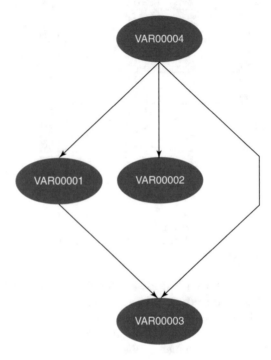

BOTTOM-UP

VAR = variable
VAR 0004 = % severe adverse drug reactions (outcome)
VAR 0003 = study size
VAR 0002 = department (1 medicine, 2 = otherwise)
VAR 0001 = year of publication of report

The percentage adverse reactions (0004) is predicted by (0001) the year of publication of report, (0002) the department, and (0003) the study size directly, and, indirectly, through the year of publication of study. This result, similarly to the above linear regression model, suggests a relationship between hospital admissions due to adverse drug reactions and the type of investigator (here called departments, either internal medicine or otherwise), but the Bayesian network, additionally, suggests, that both year of publication and study size have some predictive meaning.

14.4.2   Meta-Data from Atiqi

In the meta-data from Atiqi et al studies were assessed for hospital admissions due to severe adverse effects (Int J Clin Pharmacol Ther 2009; 47: 549–56).

VAR 1	2	3	4	5
%ADEs	Study magnitude	By Clinicians yes = 1	Elderly yes = 1	Study number
21,00	106,00	1,00	1,00	1
14,40	578,00	1,00	1,00	2
30,40	240,00	1,00	1,00	3
6,10	671,00	0,00	0,00	4
12,00	681,00	0,00	0,00	5
3,40	28411,00	1,00	0,00	6
6,60	347,00	0,00	0,00	7
3,30	8601,00	0,00	0,00	8
4,90	915,00	0,00	0,00	9
9,60	156,00	0,00	0,00	10
6,50	4093,00	0,00	0,00	11
6,50	18820,00	0,00	0,00	12
4,10	6383,00	0,00	0,00	13
4,30	2933,00	0,00	0,00	14
3,50	480,00	0,00	0,00	15
4,30	19070,00	1,00	0,00	16
12,60	2169,00	1,00	0,00	17
33,20	2261,00	0,00	1,00	18
5,60	12793,00	0,00	0,00	19
5,10	355,00	0,00	0,00	20

VAR = variable
%ADEs = percentage adverse drug effects
By clinicians = study performed by clinician investigators
Elderly = study of elderly patients

Twenty studies assessing the incidence of ADEs (adverse drug effects) were published 1995–2009, and were meta-analyzed by Atiqi et al (Int J Clin Pharmacol Ther 2009; 47: 549–56). These studies were also very heterogeneous. It was observed, that studies performed by pharmacists (0) produced lower incidences of ADEs than did the studies performed by clinicians (1). Also, the study magnitude and age of study populations per study were considered as possible causes of heterogeneity. The data are in the above table.

A multiple linear regression will be performed with percentage ADEs as outcome variable and the study magnitude, the type of investigators (pharmacist or internist), and the age of the study populations as predictors. For analysis SPSS statistical software was used. The statistical model Linear in the module Regression is required.

First enter the data in the Data View. Then

command:
Analyze....Regression....Linear....Dependent: % ADEs ....Independent(s): Study magnitude, Age, and type of investigators....click OK.

Coefficients[a]

Model		Unstandardized coefficients		Standardized coefficients	t	Sig.
		B	Std. error	Beta		
1	(Constant)	6,924	1,454		4,762	,000
	Study-magnitude	$-7.674E-5$	,000	−,071	−,500	,624
	Elderly=1	−1,393	2,885	−,075	−,483	,636
	Clinicians=1	18,932	3,359	,887	5,636	,000

[a]Dependent Variable: percentage ADEs

The above table is in the output sheets, and shows the results. After adjustment for the age of the study populations and study magnitude, the type of research group was the single and very significant predictor of the heterogeneity. Obviously, internists more often diagnosed ADEs than pharmacists did.

Next, we will perform a Bayesian network assessment, and we will use for the purpose the Knime and Weka software programs. In order for readers to perform their own analyses examples of step by step analyses are given in Machine learning in medicine a complete overview, the Chaps. 7, 70, 71, 74, Springer Heidelberg Germany, 2015, from the same authors. The software program chose this time a predictive support or top down reasoning model instead of a diagnostic support or bottom up reasoning model (see also previous section), but the results should not be different. They are given underneath.

col 3 = column 3 = type of investigator (1 = clinician, 0 = pharmacist)
col 2 = column 2 = age class (1 = elderly, 0 = younger)
col 1 = column 1 = study size
col 0 = column 0 = the % admissions to hospital due to adverse drug effects

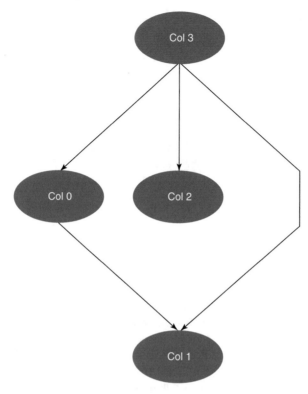

TOP-DOWN

The above graph shows that the Knime and Weka programs have chosen a top-down approach here for explaining what is going on. Again, just like with the network from the example 1, the conclusion can be: the type of investigator is an important predictor of the percentage of hospital admission due to adverse effects. And so, this example of more recent data leads to a conclusion similar to that of the first example.

The Bayesian network does not provide p-values. However, goodness of fit of the network is assessed with Akaike information index (AIC). The smaller the index, the better the network model fits the data.

$$AIC Lazarou-1\ network = -10977.9$$
$$AIC Atiqi\ network = -2080.4.$$

Both AICs were pretty small, but the Lazarou-1 was slightly smaller and thus slightly better fitted its data than the Atiqi network did. Both networks have the same conclusion: the department (= type of investigator) determines directly the amount of adverse effects.

14.4.3   Meta-Data from Lazarou-1 and Atiqi

Next a Bayesian network will be constructed from the combined data of the above
Lazarou-1 and Atiqi studies

Coefficients[a]

Model		Unstandardized coefficients		Standardized coefficients	t	Sig.
		B	Std. error	Beta		
1	(Constant)	25,985	3,262		7,965	,000
	Department	−9,514	2,023	−,629	−4,702	,000
	Study size	−8.906E − 005	,000	−.076	−,569	,573

[a]Dependent Variable: % severe

   The results of two heterogeneous meta-analyses obtained from the meta-analyses
from example 1 and 2 may provide additional power, and, possibly, new and so far
unobserved relationships. The above linear regression table shows that the type of
investigator, clinician or pharmacist, is a very significant predictor of the outcome
"% severe", meaning the % admissions to hospital admissions due to adverse drug
effects. The standardized b-value is −0.629 with a t-value of −4.702. This is very
good, but better power than the above two tests is not provided. The graph underneath shows the Bayesian network. The software has chosen again a *bottom-up*
model. The model underscored the main result from the above two networks: the
type of investigator was an independent predictor of percentages patients hospitalized for adverse drug admissions.

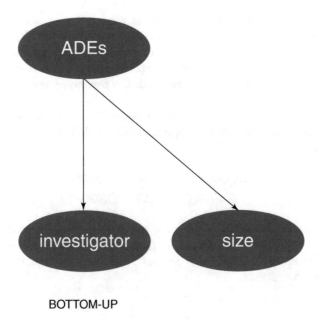

BOTTOM-UP

14.4.4 Meta-Data from Lazarou-1 and -2

Next a Bayesian network was constructed from the combined meta-data of two meta-analyses by Lazarou , one of which already assessed above. The first included patients not yet admitted to hospital, the second included patients already admitted (JAMA 1998; 279: 1200–5). The data from the second meta-analysis are below.

VAR 1	2	3	4
year of study	investigator type	study size	% admissions due to adverse effects
1996,00	2,00	450,00	5,30
1990,00	1,00	315,00	16,80
1988,00	2,00	6546,00	1,00
1987,00	1,00	686,00	6,90
1986,00	1,00	834,00	4,20
1984,00	2,00	41,00	12,20
1980,00	2,00	60,00	5,00
1977,00	2,00	442,00	6,80
1976,00	1,00	216,00	5,60
1976,00	2,00	3556,00	1,00
1974,00	1,00	6063,00	2,90
1974,00	1,00	492,00	3,30
1874,00	1,00	555,00	1,80
1974,00	1,00	1025,00	3,00
1974,00	1,00	1193,00	5,60
1974,00	1,00	2065,00	2,00
1973,00	2,00	658,00	2,90
1970,00	1,00	939,00	5,10
1967,00	1,00	267,00	4,50
1966,00	1,00	714,00	3,90
1966,00	1,00	900,00	1,70

VAR = variable
investigator type = department internal medicine or otherwise
% admissions due to adverse effects = percentage of all admissions

Coefficients[a]

Model		Unstandardized coefficients		Standardized coefficients	t	Sig.
		B	Std. error	Beta		
1	(Constant)	−95,518	101,603		−,940	,354
	Year of study	,054	,052	,180	1,048	,302
	Department	−3,247	2,040	−,275	−1,591	,121
	Study size	,000	,000	,057	,346	,732

[a]Dependent Variable: % severe

Lazarou (JAMA 1998; 279: 1200–5) provided an additional set of studies providing information about studies who assessed adverse drug reactions in patients
already admitted to hospital. The above table provides a linear regression of both the
patients admitted because of adverse drug reactions, and those already in hospital
with adverse drug reactions. They included 39 studies (Lazarou JAMA 1998; 279:
1202) of percentages of hospitalized patients with adverse drug reactions.

The above table shows that none of the predictors of % severe (percentage of
patients in hospital with adverse drug reactions) were statistically significant, a
pretty disappointing result. Bayesian network models were constructed using the
above KNIME and WEKA software once more.

It suggested, that investigator type predicted the percentage of patients hospitalized for adverse drug reactions, and was, thus, again entirely in agreement with the
results of the above three Bayesian networks. We should add that, although p-values
were not provided by the software, the consistency of the results was, obviously,
very good. If you don't have additional data files, another way of assessing consistency of the results of the networks is to do some kind of cross validation to assess
the reliability of the network.

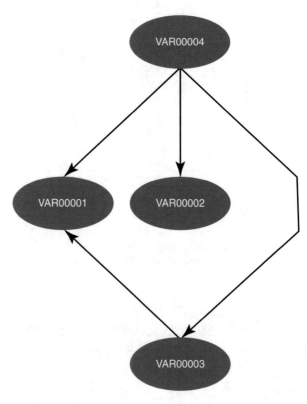

BOTTOM-UP

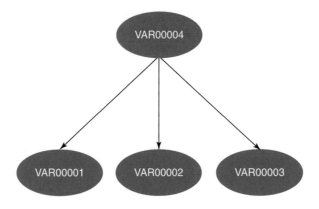

BOTTOM-UP

The above two networks included the Lazarou-1 and -2 meta-data, and were thus partly based on the same data as those of the former networks is different from the former. Which of networks performs best? Akaike information (AIC) indexes (otherwise called Bayesian information (BIC) criteria) are used for assessment. Briefly, it is a goodness of fit test, calculated from the difference between the numbers of parameters minus their likelihood score. The smaller the Akaike information index, the better the fit of the model.

$$\text{AIC Lazarou-1 network} = -10977.9$$
$$\text{AIC Atiqi network} = -2080.4$$
$$\text{AIC Lazarou-1 and-2 upper graph} = -6652.3$$
$$\text{AIC Lazarou-1 and-2 lower graph} = -37.7$$

This would mean that the first of the two Lazarou-1 and -2 networks provided a much better fit for the data given than did the latter. As compared to the other networks, overall the Lazarou-1 has provided the best fit network. All of the five networks constructed have largely the same conclusions. The department (= type of investigator) determines directly the amount of adverse effects in all of them.

14.4.5   *Discussion*

Three previously published meta-analyses assessing the effect of various predictors on the frequency of iatrogenic hospital admissions were re-analyzed separately and in combination. Five different networks were produced by the Konstanz Information Miner (Knime). One network provided a much better fit for the data than the other.

In the past few years the network methodology has also been used as a method for synthesizing information from a network of trials addressing the same question but involving different interventions (Mills et al., JAMA 2012; 308: 1246–53, and Cipriani et al., Ann Intern Med 2013; 159: 130–7). The key assumption with any type of network meta-analysis is, of course, the exchangeability assumption: patient and study characteristics of studies in the meta-analysis must be similar enough to be comparable. The exchangeability assumption can sometimes be tested, but this is virtually always hard to do. E.g., a trial with three treatment arms A versus B versus C, should have the same effects of A versus C and B versus C as separate trials of two treatment arms should have. Currently, Extended Bucher networks (Song et al, BMJ 2011; 343: d4909) and Lumley networks (Stat Med 2002; 21: 2313–24) can cover for more complex networks with contrast coefficients adding up to one.

14.5   Bayesian Networks in Ensembled Procedures

14.5.1   Example

A 200 patients' data file includes 11 variables consistent of patients' laboratory values and their subsequent outcome (death or alive). Only the first 12 patients are shown underneath. The entire data file is in extras.springer.com, and is entitled "chap14-3".

Death	ggt	asat	alat	bili	ureum	creat	c-clear	esr	crp	leucos
,00	20,00	23,00	34,00	2,00	3,40	89,00	−111,00	2,00	2,00	5,00
,00	14,00	21,00	33,00	3,00	2,00	67,00	−112,00	7,00	3,00	6,00
,00	30,00	35,00	32,00	4,00	5,60	58,00	−116,00	8,00	4,00	4,00
,00	35,00	34,00	40,00	4,00	6,00	76,00	−110,00	6,00	5,00	7,00
,00	23,00	33,00	22,00	4,00	6,10	95,00	−120,00	9,00	6,00	6,00
,00	26,00	31,00	24,00	3,00	5,40	78,00	−132,00	8,00	4,00	8,00
,00	15,00	29,00	26,00	2,00	5,30	47,00	−120,00	12,00	5,00	5,00
,00	13,00	26,00	24,00	1,00	6,30	65,00	−132,00	13,00	6,00	6,00
,00	26,00	27,00	27,00	4,00	6,00	97,00	−112,00	14,00	6,00	7,00
,00	34,00	25,00	13,00	3,00	4,00	67,00	−125,00	15,00	7,00	6,00
,00	32,00	26,00	24,00	3,00	3,60	58,00	−110,00	13,00	8,00	6,00
,00	21,00	13,00	15,00	3,00	3,60	69,00	−102,00	12,00	2,00	4,00

death = death yes no (0 = no)
ggt = gamma glutamyl transferase (u/l)
asat = aspartate aminotransferase (u/l)
alat = alanine aminotransferase (u/l)
bili = bilirubine (micromol/l)
ureum = ureum (mmol/l)
creat= creatinine (mmicromol/l)
c-clear = creatinine clearance (ml/min)
esr = erythrocyte sedimentation rate (mm)
crp = c-reactive protein (mg/l)
leucos = leucocyte count (.10^9/l)

14.5.2 Step 1 Open SPSS Modeler (Sect. 14.2)

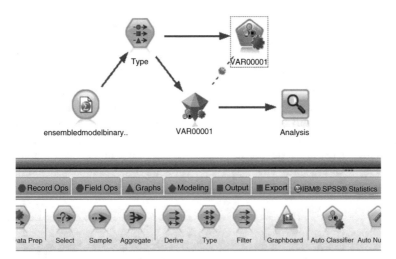

14.5.3 Step 2 the Statistics File Node

The canvas is, initially, blank, and above is given a screen view of the completed ensembled model which we are going to build. First, in the palettes at the bottom of the screen full of nodes, look and find the **Statistics File node**, and drag it to the canvas, pressing the mouse left side. Double-click on this node….Import file: browse and enter the file entitled "chap14-2" ….click OK. The graph below shows, that the data file is open for analysis.

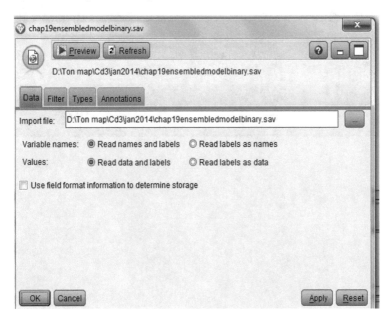

14.5.4 Step 3 the Type Node

In the palette at the bottom of screen find Type node and drag to the canvas....
right-click on the Statistics File node....a Connect symbol comes up....click on
the Type node....an arrow is displayed....double-click on the Type Node....after a
second or two the underneath graph with information from the Type node is
observed. Type nodes are used to access the properties of the variables (often
called fields here) like type, role, unit etc. in the data file. As shown below, 10
predictor variables (all of them continuous) are appropriately set. However, VAR
00001 (death) is the outcome (= target) variable, and is binary. Click in the row
of variable VAR00001 on the measurement column and replace "Continuous"
with "Flag". Click Apply and OK. The underneath figure is removed and the canvas is displayed again.

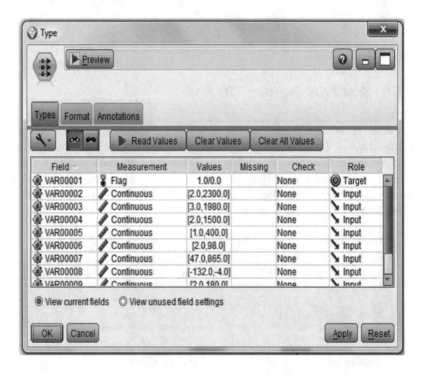

14.5.5   Step 4 the Auto Classifier Node

Now, click the Auto Classifier node and drag to the canvas, and connect with the Type node using the above connect-procedure. Click the Auto Classifier node, and the underneath graph comes up....now click Model....select Lift as Rank model of the various analysis models used.... the additional manoeuvres are as indicated below....in Numbers of models to use: type the number 4.

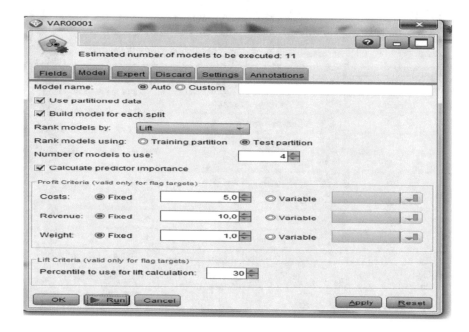

14.5.6   Step 5 the Expert Tab

Then click the Expert tab. It is shown below. Out of 11 statistical models the four best fit ones are selected by SPSS Modeler for constructing an ensembled model.

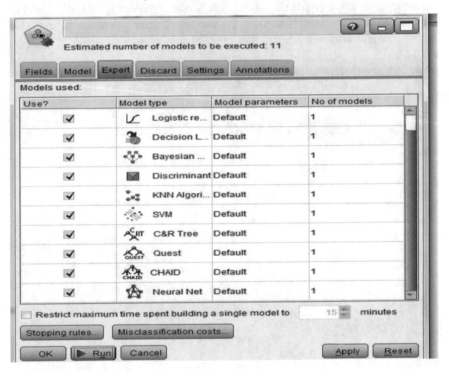

The 11 statistical analysis methods for a flag target (= binary outcome) include:

1/ C5.0 decision tree (C5.0)
2/ Logistic regression (Logist r…)
3/ Decision list (Decision….)
4/ Bayesian network (Bayesian….)
5/ Discriminant analysis (Discriminant)
6/ K nearest neighbors algorithm (KNN Alg…)
7/ Support vector machine (SVM)
8/ Classification and regression tree (C&R Tree)
9/ Quest decision tree (Quest Tr….)
10/ Chi square automatic interaction detection (CHAID Tree)
11/ Neural network (Neural Net)

14.5.7   Step 6 the Settings Tab

In the above graph click the Settings tab….click the Run button….now a gold nugget is placed on the canvas….click the gold nugget….the model created is shown below.

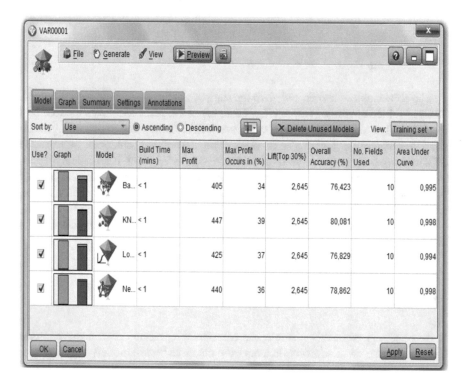

The overall accuracies (%) of the four best fit models are over 0.8, and are, thus, pretty good. We will now perform the ensembled procedure.

14.5.8   Step 7 the Analysis Node

Find in the palettes at the bottom of the screen the Analysis node and drag it to the canvas. With above connect procedure connect it with the gold nugget….click the Analysis node.

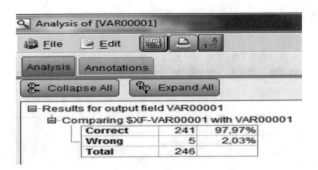

The above table is shown and gives the statistics of the ensembled model created. The ensembled outcome is the average accuracy of the accuracies from the four best fit statistical models. In order to prevent overstated certainty due to overfitting, bootstrap aggregating ("bagging") is used. The ensembled outcome (named the $XR-outcome) is compared with the outcomes of the four best fit statistical models, namely, Bayesian network, k Nearest Neighbor clustering, Logistic regression, and Neural network. The ensembled accuracy (97.97%) is much larger than the accuracies of the four best fit models (76.423, 80,081, 76,829, and 78,862), and, so, ensembled procedures make sense because they provide increased precision in the analysis.

14.5.9   Discussion

In the results given in this example, the ensembled regression coefficients is larger (0.859) than the correlation coefficients from the three best fit models (0.854, 0.836, 0.821), and so ensembled procedures make sense because they can provide increased precision in the analysis.

SPSS Modeler is a software program entirely distinct from SPSS statistical software, though it uses most if not all of the calculus methods of it. It is a standard software package particularly used by market analysts, but as shown can perfectly well be applied for exploratory purposes in medical research.

14.6   Conclusion

A Bayesian network (BN) is a tool to describe and analyze multivariate distributions. The tool is member of the family of probabilistic graphical models. Graphical models in general, and Bayesian networks too, have been proposed especially to deal with complex data (-analysis), and with an eye towards causal interpretations. This is achieved by combining graph theory, particularly path analysis and path statistics, probability theory, statistics and computer science. Bayesian networks have been used in many different fields, for instance, in the Microsoft Windows system and the NASA mission control. In biomedicine the main applications seems to be in expert systems, in bioinformatics applications in genetics, and in identifying gene-regulatory networks. In biomedicine the main applications are in expert systems, in bioinformatics applications in genetics, and in identifying gene-regulatory networks, with a particular eye towards causal relationships. This chapter assesses whether a best fit Bayesian network can be used:

1. for cause effect modeling in surveys,
2. for cause effect modeling in clinical trials,
3. for analyzing meta-data,
4. in ensembled procedures.

Step by step analyses of data examples are described using the respective software programs: (1) Knime (Konstanz Information Miner), (2) Matlab Bayes Net Toolbox, (3) Knime and Weka (Waikato environment for knowledge analysis software), and (4) SPSS Modeler.

We conclude that the graphical display of Bayesian networks has been adopted by many disciplines, to describe causal pathways. The graphical tools have proved to be appealing in many applied fields, but they are somewhat problematic in biomedicine, because confounding and interaction effects are often involved. Nonetheless, Bayesian networks are very efficient to describe multivariate distributions in clinical surveys, clinical trials, clinical meta-analyses, and ensemble procedures. The structure makes inferences from Bayesian networks robust, reduces variances of estimated parameters, and is also robust against overfitting.

Suggested Reading[1,2]

Statistics applied to clinical studies 5th edition, 2012,
Machine learning in medicine a complete overview, 2015,
SPSS for starters and 2nd levelers 2nd edition, 2015,
Clinical data analysis on a pocket calculator 2nd edition, 2016,
Understanding clinical data analysis from published research, 2016,
Modern Meta-analysis, 2017,
Regression Analysis in Clinical Research, 2018.

---

[1] To readers requesting more background, theoretical and mathematical information of computations given, several textbooks complementary to the current production and written by the same authors are available.

[2] All of them have been written by the same authors, and they have been edited by Springer Heidelberg Germany.

Summary

Chapter 1

With Bayesian statistics there is no traditional null (H0) and alternative hypothesis (H1) like there is with standard null hypothesis testing. Instead there is a standardized likelihood distribution to assess whether a new treatment is better or worse than control.

The term odds, otherwise called the ratio of [the chance of having a disease]/ [chance of having no disease], plays a key role not only in logistic regressions and Cox regressions, but also in traditional Bayes statistical analyses as post-test odds and pre-test odds, where post-test odds = prior-test odds x likelihood ratio.

Modern Bayes does not work with normal distributions, but likelihood distributions, that are approximated differently. The traditional Bayes factor is not the area under the curve (AUC) of a likelihood distribution curve, but, rather, the ratio of the AUCs of two likelihood distributions. We should add, that the ratio of two odds values, has often been named Bayes factor with traditional Bayesian statistics, but with modern Bayesian statistics the Bayes factors are mostly based on the ratios of two likelihood distributions.

In the past the non exact intuitive definition of the prior was the Achilles heal of Bayes. Fortunately, the intuitive prior and the posterior odds have been replaced with more exact likelihood distributions and interpretations based on intervals of uncertainty.

Differences between traditional and Bayesian Statistics may include.

1. A better underlying structure of the alternative hypothesis H1 and the null hypothesis H0 may be provided.
2. Bayesian tests work with 95% credible intervals that are usually somewhat wider and this may reduce the chance of statistical significances with little clinical relevance.
3. Maximal likelihoods of likelihood distributions are not always identical to the mean effect of traditional tests, and this may be fine, because biological

© Springer International Publishing AG, part of Springer Nature 2018

T. J. Cleophas, A. H. Zwinderman, *Modern Bayesian Statistics in Clinical Research*,
https://doi.org/10.1007/978-3-319-92747-3

likelihoods may better fit biological questions than numerical means of non-representative subgroups do.

4. Bayes uses ratios of likelihood distributions rather than ratios of Gaussian distributions, which are notorious for ill data fit.

5. Bayesian integral computations are very advanced, and, therefore, give optimal precisions of complex functions, and better so than traditional multiple mean calculations of non representative subsamples do.

6. With Bayesian testing type I (alpha) and II (beta) errors need not being taken into account.

Chapter 2

In clinical research where the base rate for a disease is very low and the diagnostic test is far from perfect, there will be a pretty high probability of a positive result that is false positive. Traditional Bayesian statistics uses the ratios of posterior and prior test odds, where the odds is again the ratio of patients being true positive (having some disease) and that of being true negative (having none disease). The methodology has been traditionally used for three main purposes:

1. diagnostic testing,
2. genetic data analyses,
3. finding the probability in drug trials that a new drug will really work.

The current chapter will review the three purposes. We will give examples, including examples of populations with

rare diseases,
more common,
common,
very common like a genetic disease with 50% gene carrier ship,
very common with 75% prevalence.

Also examples will be given of Bayesian statistics applied for genetic data analysis, and for analyzing drug trials with type I and type II errors assessed in the form of Bayesian prior probability estimates.

Chapter 3

In studies with one sample continuous data a single outcome per patient is usually compared to zero.

Instead of t-test also a Bayesian one sample normal test is possible. A one sample t-test of a hypertension study provided a result significantly different from zero at t = 2.429, p = 0.038. A Bayesian one sample t-test provided support in favor of the above t-test with a Bayes factor of 0.506. The 95% confidence intervals of (1) the traditional test, (2) the Bayesian test, and (3) the bootstrap t-test were respectively

0.1165–3.2835
−0.1769 to 3.5769
0.4000–2.9000.

Therefore, some overfitting cannot be ruled out. We conclude that in this chapter the Bayes factor is a better test statistic than the traditional p-value is.

Chapter 4

In studies with one sample of binomial data (yes no data) the z-test is pretty much traditionally used for analysis.

Instead of a z-test also a Bayesian one sample binomial test is possible. A one sample z-test of a hypertension study provided a z-value of 5.5545 and a p-value < 0.001.

A Bayesian one sample binomial test provided less support in favor of the above z-test with a Bayes factor (BF) of only 1.0. Nonetheless, as BFs run from ∞ to 0.0 and p-values run from 1.0 to 0.0, the Bayesian and traditional statistics are very well compatible with one another.

The 95% confidence intervals of the Bayesian and traditional tests of

[0.256–0.499], and
[0.2327–0.4945]

were pretty similar, although the Bayesian interval was a bit wider. Therefore, some overfitting of the Bayesian statistics could not be ruled out.

Chapter 5

In studies with paired samples of continuous data the mean difference is usually compared to zero. Instead of a paired t-test also a Bayesian analysis on the mean difference is possible. A traditional paired t-test of two treatment modalities on hours of sleep provided a significant difference with t = 3.184, p-value = 0.011. A Bayesian paired t-test provided support in favor of the traditional test with a Bayes factor of 0.178. The 95% confidence intervals of (1) traditional, (2) Bayesian and (3) bootstrap tests were respectively:

between 0.51517 and 3.04483,
between 0.2809 and 3.2791,
between 0.76025 and 2.8400.

The traditional t-test confidence interval was wider than the bootstraps t-test confidence interval, while the Bayesian 95% credible interval is the widest. Some overfitting in the traditional and Bayesian intervals can not be ruled out, and, in the Bayesian, this may be more so than in the traditional. Nonetheless, the amount of overfitting is limited with confidence intervals between $\approx$2.3 and $\approx$2.8.

Chapter 6

In studies with two unpaired samples of continuous data the difference of the two means and their pooled standard error is usually compared to zero. Instead of an unpaired t-test also a Bayesian analysis on the difference of two group means is possible. A traditional unpaired t-test of parallel group study provided a statistically significantly difference in treatment efficacy with t = -3.558, p-value = 0.002. A Bayesian unpaired t-test provided support in favor of the traditional test with a Bayes factor of 0.056. The robustness was assessed.

1. Bootstraps unpaired t-test 95% confidence interval	-2.61536 to -0.71752
2. Bayesian unpaired t-test 95% credible interval	-2.8098 to -0.6302
3. Gaussian unpaired t-test 95% confidence interval	-2.73557 to -0.79443

Obviously the 95% confidence interval of the bootstraps t-test was closer to the traditional Gaussian t-test than it was to the Bayesian t-test. Under the assumption that bootstrap sampling is entirely without overfitting, this would be an argument of overfitting of the Bayesian t-test and an argument in favor of the traditional Gaussian approach. However, with an informed prior this was less a problem.

Chapter 7

In studies with two unpaired samples of continuous data as outcome and a binary predictor like treatment modality the difference of the two means and their pooled standard error is usually compared to zero. Instead of the above tests a Bayesian regression analysis is possible.

A traditional regression analysis with a single binary predictor provided a linear correlation coefficient of 0.643, p-value = 0.002, and a linear regression coefficient of -1.720, t = -3.558, p-value = 0.002. A Bayesian regression of these data did not compute "supporting null versus alternative hypothesis" but, in contrast, the other ways around, and it provided support in favor of the traditional test with a Bayes factor of 17.329.

A traditional regression analysis with multiple binary predictors provided a linear correlation coefficient of 0.669, p-value = 0.021, and only one significant linear regression coefficients of −1.642, t = −3.223, p-value = 0.005. A Bayesian regression of these data did again not compute "supporting null versus alternative hypothesis" but, in contrast, the other ways around, and it provided support in favor of the traditional test with a Bayes factor of 1.626.

A traditional regression analysis with a single continuous predictor provided a linear correlation coefficient of 0.975, p-value = 0.000, and a linear regression coefficient of 0.093, t = 18.443, p-value = 0.000. A Bayesian regression of these data again did not compute "supporting null versus alternative hypothesis" but, in contrast, the other ways around, and it provided support in favor of the traditional test with a Bayes factor of 2.284[10].

A disadvantage of Bayesian analysis may be an increased risk of overfitting, but in the regression examples in this chapter this was virtually not observed.

Chapter 8

In studies with two unpaired samples of continuous data as outcome and a binary predictor like treatment modality unpaired t-tests are usually applied. With three or more unpaired samples traditional t-tests are impossible, and analysis of variance (anova) must be applied. Instead of a traditional Anova a Bayesian Anova is possible. A traditional analysis of variance with three treatment modalities as predictor provided a Fisher (F) statistic of 14.110, p-value = 0.0001. A Bayesian analysis of variance of these data did not compute "supporting null versus alternative hypothesis" but, in contrast, the other ways around, and it provided support in favor of the traditional test with a Bayes factor of 389.479. The 95% credible intervals gave an impression about the widths of the likelihood distributions.

	95% confidence interval	95% credible interval
Group 0.0	6.3537–7.5063	6.179–7.681
Group 1.0	4.2807–6.1393	4.459–5.961
Group 3.0	3.2807–5.1393	3.459–4.961

The group 0 credible interval was a bit wider than the traditional 95% confidence interval was. The groups 2 and 3 credible intervals were a bit narrower. Obviously, group 0 provided the best likelihood in favor of the alternative hypothesis H1.

The Bayes factor (BF) in this example of 389.479 gave very strong support of the alternative hypothesis, and was compatible with the p-value of <0.0001 as obtained from the traditional one way anova.

Chapter 9

In studies with both a binary outcome (for example event yes/no) and binary predictor variable (for example treatment group 1 or 2) for traditional analysis, a 2×2 interaction matrix can be drawn with the predictor in two rows and the outcome in two columns. Instead of a 2×2 chi-square test also a Bayesian loglinear regression is possible. The mathematical model of a linear regression and loglinear regression are respectively

$$y = a + bx, \text{and}$$
$$\log y = a + bx,$$

where log is usually the natural logarithm of the variable y. A traditional 2×2 analysis provided a chi-square value of 5.304, with a p-value 0.021. The null hypothesis of no difference between two treatment groups could be rejected. A Bayesian loglinear regression provided support in favor of the traditional test with a Bayes factor (BF) of 0.161. The BF was slightly closer to 0.0 (or very small) than the p-value of 0.021 was to 0.0, and, so, the BF seemed to provide a slightly better test statistic than the p-value did. The confidence intervals of three approaches are underneath.

1. Gaussian 95% confidence interval 0.148 and 2.624
2. Bootstrap 95% confidence interval 0.176 and 3.043
3. Bayesian 95% credible interval 0.176 and 2.528.

Obviously, the Gaussian confidence interval, the bootstrap confidence interval, and the Bayesian credible interval had very much similarly sized intervals. Overfitting was not obvious.

Chapter 10

Poisson analysis is adequate for studies where event rate per patient per period of exposure is used as main outcome. Unlike normal distributions, the Poisson distribution depends on just one parameter which is the mean number of events per person per period of time. Its standard error equals $\sqrt{\text{mean}}$.

Instead of a traditional Poisson rate test also a Bayesian Poison rate test one sample normal test is possible.

A traditional Poisson regression using the generalized linear models module in SPSS statistical software provided a mean event rate of 6.120 with a 95% confidence interval 5.463–6.862, significantly different from zero at p-value = 0.000, goodness of fit with a Bayesian Information Criterion of 500.637.

A Bayesian Poisson rate analysis provided support in favor of the traditional test with a Bayes factor of 0.061. The credible interval of the Bayesian analysis was hardly different from that of the traditional model, namely between 5.28 and 6.60.

Chapter 11

In studies with two continuous variables usually named the x-values and y-values a linear relation between the two variables can be assessed with the help of the Pearson correlation coefficient R. R is a measure of strength of association, and varies from −1 to +1. Instead of a traditional Pearson correlation analysis a Bayesian analysis of linear correlation is possible.

A traditional analysis of Pearson linear correlation analysis provided an r-value of 0.483 with an F statistic of 10047, p-value 0.003. A Bayesian Analysis of Pearson linear correlation provided support in favor of the traditional test with a Bayes factor of 0.105.

The maximum of the posterior likelihood distribution was 0.478 with 95% credible interval

$$0.183 \text{ to } 0.685.$$

This was less wide than the 95% confidence interval of the traditional Pearson linear correlation which was

$$0.483 \pm 2 \times \left[\left(4.83 \times 0.553 \right) / 0.174 \right] =$$
$$0.483 \pm 2 \times 0.1535 =$$
$$\text{between } 0.176 \text{ and } 0.790.$$

Thus, the Bayesian analysis provided slightly better statistics than did the traditional Pearson correlation analysis.

Chapter 12

Markov chain Monte Carlo (MCMC) procedures can be laid out as Bayesian tests. The Bayesian prior likelihood distribution of MCMC procedures could, for example, be a data file with missing data. The posterior likelihood distribution is based on the prior plus the MCMC computed imputation values. In a 500 patient multiple variables model with missing data five MCMC imputed models were produced with the help of the multiple imputations module in SPSS statistical software. The correlation coefficients of the predictor versus outcome values in the original data and those of five MCMC imputed models were respectively

0.533
0.596
0.567
0.594
0.586
0.580.

The Bayes factors of the Bayesian analyses of the above imputated models were respectively

1.187963
2.671638
1.518048
2.537739
2.142738
1.90718.

We conclude that both the traditional correlation coefficients of the imputated models and their Bayes factors were consistently robuster. However, the magnitudes of the Bayes factors increased over 100%, while the magnitudes of the traditional correlation coefficients increased by 8% at best.

Chapter 13

The current search for causal relationships with Bayesian structural equation modelings will be addressed in this chapter as an example where Bayesian methodologies successfully helped fostering the deepest enigma of mankind, the proof of causality.

A Bayesian equation looks much like a simple path analysis, and, can, actually, be analyzed similarly. The underneath equations give examples of this (Var = variable):

prior likelihood distribution × Bayes factor = posterior likelihood distribution

path statistic 1 × path statistic 2 = effect of Var 1 through Var 2 on Var 3.

Multistep regressions are the basis of path analysis, and path analysis is the basis of Bayesian networks, using structural equation modeling (SEM). They can be visualized with DAGs (directed acyclic graphs), with arrows meant to indicate causality. If SEMs include

latent factors (unmeasured variables inferred from measured variables) as predictors, we will call it:

factor analysis if unsupervised (i.e., no dependent variable);
partial least squares if supervised;
discriminant analysis if like the above two but including a grouping variable.

manifest factors (variables), we will call it:

multistage regressions which might include flawed predictors, given pejorative names, like problematic predictors, multicollinear predictors, indirect predictors.

Bayesian networks do not necessarily use traditional Bayesian statistics, i.e., posterior and prior odds. Instead they may use the methodologies of more modern Bayesian statistics, i.e., conditional and marginal probability distributions (running from 0 to 1), and likelihood distributions (even running from 0 to ∞).

Chapter 14

A Bayesian network (BN) is a tool to describe and analyze multivariate distributions. In biomedicine the main applications are in expert systems, in bioinformatics applications in genetics, and in identifying gene-regulatory networks, with a particular eye towards causal relationships. This chapter is to assess whether a best fit Bayesian network can be used:

1. for cause effect modeling in surveys,
2. for cause effect modeling in clinical trials,
3. for analyzing meta-data,
4. in ensembled procedures.

Step by step analyses of data examples are described. Analyses were performed with the help of the underneath respective software programs:

1. Knime (Konstanz Information Miner),
2. Matlab Bayes Net Toolbox,
3. Knime and Weka (Waikato environment for knowledge analysis software),
4. SPSS Modeler.

We come to conclude that the graphical display of Bayesian networks has been adopted very widely, for instance, by biomolecular scientists to describe pathogenetic, metabolic, and other causal pathways. The graphical tools have proved to be appealing in every applied field, but they are somewhat problematic in biomedicine, because confounding and interaction effects are often involved. Nonetheless, Bayesian networks are very efficient to describe multivariate distributions. The structure makes inferences from Bayesian networks robust, reduces variances of estimated parameters, and is also robust against overfitting.

Index

© Springer International Publishing AG, part of Springer Nature 2018
T. J. Cleophas, A. H. Zwinderman, *Modern Bayesian Statistics in Clinical Research*,
https://doi.org/10.1007/978-3-319-92747-3

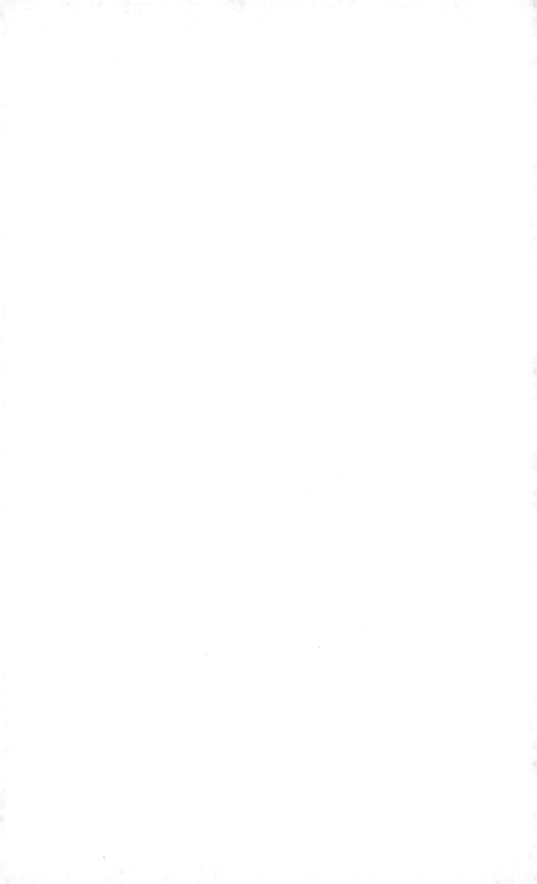

Printed in the United States
By Bookmasters